# One Life
# at a Time

# One Life at a Time

## AN AMERICAN DOCTOR'S
## MEMOIR of AIDS
## in BOTSWANA

## Daniel Baxter

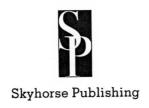

Skyhorse Publishing

Skyhorse Publishing books may be purchased in bulk at special discounts for sales promotion, corporate gifts, fund-raising, or educational purposes. Special editions can also be created to specifications. For details, contact the Special Sales Department, Skyhorse Publishing, 307 West 36th Street, 11th Floor, New York, NY 10018 or info@skyhorsepublishing.com.

Skyhorse® and Skyhorse Publishing® are registered trademarks of Skyhorse Publishing, Inc.®, a Delaware corporation.

Visit our website at www.skyhorsepublishing.com.

10 9 8 7 6 5 4 3 2 1

Library of Congress Cataloging-in-Publication Data is available on file.

Cover design by Russell Stark

Print ISBN: 978-1-5107-3576-7
Ebook ISBN: 978-1-5107-3577-4

*To Eleanor, John, Daniel, Jack, and my many patients, students, and colleagues in Botswana*

# Contents

# Acknowledgements

This book has many "authors:" my friends and colleagues in Botswana, my many KITSO students, the medical students and residents at Princess Marina Hospital, and, above all, the countless patients I had the privilege of caring for during my eight-and-a-half years in Botswana. I am also indebted to the people and government of Botswana and the African Comprehensive HIV/AIDS Partnerships for allowing me the opportunity to work with the country's HIV/AIDS Treatment Programme, the first in Africa and salvation for over 100,000 people with HIV/AIDS.

Andrea Nattrass of Pan Macmillan South Africa had the courage and foresight to take on my book, and to shepherd it through the publishing process. Andrea cares deeply about how AIDS has affected not just her native South Africa, but also the entire continent. I am also indebted to Russell Martin for editing and polishing my book for publication in sub-Saharan Africa. My gratitude to them knows no bounds.

Skyhorse Publishing likewise recognized the importance of my book and accepted it for release in North America. Tony Lyons,

Andrew Geller, and Mark Gompertz have provided invaluable help in guiding it through the publishing process in New York.

I am also very grateful for the efforts of my agent, Andrew Stuart, the unstinting support of Bob Weil, and the unconditional love of my wonderful family.

# Preface

The evening before I left New York City for Botswana in 2002, my friend Bob invited me to dinner with two acquaintances of his, a famous cardiothoracic surgeon and his wife, a well-known literary agent. They were the quintessential New York "power couple," and the restaurant, Cipriani, was well suited to their cosmopolitan tastes. The surgeon was interested in my decision to move to Botswana, to help its recently launched HIV/AIDS Treatment Programme. He wanted to know why I was doing it, why I was leaving a high-profile job as medical director of a large community health center. Unlike most other people when they learned about my plans, he didn't gush and exclaim how wonderful I was to do such a thing. Rather, he seemed perplexed, even disturbed at my plans. Although I had always wanted to work in a developing country, I suddenly found myself tongue-tied, unable to articulate my motivations clearly. I was annoyed with his questioning what I thought was the fundamental goodness of helping people less advantaged than myself. Flustered, I yammered on about how people in Botswana had the same hopes and fears about suffering as we Americans had, and how I wanted to experience for myself the universality of such feelings. Without the slightest trace of superiority—he sounded measured and thoughtful—the surgeon replied, "I'm not so sure about that." Uncomfortable at my inability to state my motivations for moving to Botswana, I changed the subject.

Although I was unaware of it at the time, my glib answer and the surgeon's skeptical reply perfectly framed the illusions that would come crashing down soon after my arrival in Botswana. Only many years later did I fully understand my dinner companion's wisdom in challenging the reason I gave for going to Botswana.

This book is an account of my own journey through one of the great human struggles of the early twenty-first century: AIDS in Africa. I had gone to Botswana thinking I had nothing substantial to learn, especially about myself. But soon after I arrived with all of my seemingly good—and often misguided—intentions, Africa punctured my arrogance, exposing my inadequacy and selfishness. But Africa's time and space eventually gave me solace, and allowed me to soldier on, transforming my naive altruism into something more honest and substantial.

In the stories that follow, the patients' names have been changed, and to preserve confidentiality further, various details and other names have sometimes been altered. Nonetheless, the pages that follow faithfully capture the life-changing experiences of my sojourn with fellow sufferers in Botswana.

# Prologue

Long considered a tourist destination for watching wild animals, Botswana has always been a place most Americans have heard about but few can pinpoint on a map. Indeed, when I was first contacted about a job there in 2002, I had to pretend I knew where it was, before quickly searching for it online. The first internet entry I found explained why Botswana had always been so easy to overlook: it's the size of France, landlocked, and mostly desert—the Kalahari comprises 70 percent of it—and it's one of the most sparsely populated countries in the world. Its 1.6 million people are a million less than the population of Brooklyn. Initially, the article was at best routine, and reminded me of my soporific eighth-grade geography class in Ohio so many years ago. Routine, that is, until the very end, where a brief paragraph mentioned the AIDS epidemic unfolding there: no less than 24 percent of Botswana's people were reported to be infected already with HIV, then the highest rate in the world after Swaziland, a smaller country to the south. Life expectancy was projected to plunge by twenty to thirty years by mid-decade. I already knew that all of sub-Saharan

Africa was in the crosshairs of the HIV epidemic, but as an AIDS doctor in New York City, I should have known these sobering statistics without the help of Wikipedia. Being slightly hermetic, an African version of Switzerland, somehow hadn't spared Botswana from the plague.

Sight unseen, I immediately accepted the job.

However, geography books and online articles rarely can capture the real sense of a place, especially Botswana, where I soon realized that one had to look upward to the heavens to counter the very distinct plainness—and too often a mantle of sadness—at ground level below. The blueness of the Botswana sky is unique, a hue unlike any other in the world. Adjectives like limpid, crystalline, and cerulean come to mind, but even these words cannot convey the awesome blue infinitude of the firmament overhead. This immensity of time and space can easily overwhelm someone unaccustomed to it. But for me the predictable mid-afternoon advent of Botswana's clouds added welcome texture and reassuring dimension to the endless expanse of sky.

As I would discover, Botswana's cumulus clouds were unfailingly exuberant, fat, if not downright bodacious, unlike the smudged cirrus variety usually brooding over the skyline of New York City. An endless armada of fluffy galleons floating serenely across the sky, at times so close to earth you felt you could almost touch them, Botswana's clouds seemed unconcerned with the desperate struggles for survival playing out beneath them, struggles in which I soon found myself, both physically and existentially, enmeshed. Later in the afternoon, these frigates would coalesce into thunderhead behemoths of biblical proportions, stretching to all corners of the compass, as if poised to do combat against one another. But at sunset, they would rapidly fade into a flat, pinkish haze, to make way for the moon and star-bejeweled sky of night. At dusk I would often sit out alone on my porch, reflecting on the patients I had seen that day . . .

*Eunice, a Holy Cross Hospice patient who needed a residency permit so she could continue her HIV treatment in Botswana and not be deported to her native Zimbabwe . . . doctors are supposed to be honest and truthful, but what if being truthful would result in irreparable harm? . . .*

*Mercy, the clinic nurse who had "a great pain in my heart" over unwelcome news, quietly divulging her anguished decision so her partner wouldn't abandon her and her five children . . . and as with so many of my patients, she concluded her sad story with "But God is good" . . .*

*The thirty-two-year-old prisoner, essentially a gasping skeleton, gingerly carried into the clinic by his worried cellmate, and the terrified gaze of their robust guard, who seemed to see his own fate from the contagion wracking his charge . . .*

*"No Fear," a rude guy at my gym, at first my nemesis and then my ex-nemesis, whose gradual descent was halted by my gruffly shouting out to him one day . . .*

*Godwill, a frightened illegal Zimbabwean with severe shingles and AIDS, sheltered by his church in the rural Kalahari, and cared for by a clinic nurse, who, breaking government rules concerning noncitizens, answered to a higher authority . . .*

There would be patients I feared I might have harmed . . .

*Comfort, an emaciated ten-year-old girl in the capital's slum . . . had my overly attentive care—and hubris—hastened her demise? . . .*

*Polite, my maid . . . did my standoffish reticence, borne of America's obsession about HIV confidentiality, cause the turmoil she was enduring, making her fear that she was "killing" her newborn baby boy? . . .*

And there were those whose extremity, for reasons I could never fully articulate, transfixed me, evoking my deepest hopes and fears . . .

*Precious, a Holy Cross Hospice patient teetering on the edge of the abyss, alone in her Old Naledi hovel—I really, really wanted her to make it, yet was terrified that my intense hopes would provoke the indifferent fates to strike her down . . . she should have been "just another AIDS patient" . . .*

*Grace, panting into her oxygen mask as her pneumonia threatened to pull her down . . . she seemed fearful of leaving this earth, whereas her ward-mate Charity, also with a serious pneumonia, didn't seem to care if she recovered or died . . .*

*Isaac, my fourteen year old slowly sliding into the grave as he languished in Marina Hospital, pining to return to his sister in their remote village in the Kalahari . . . his suffering evoked both nothing and everything from me . . . you really can't tell a 14 year-old he's dying from AIDS . . .*

*Dolly, twenty years old, raped by her pastor at age thirteen, dying alone at Marina, who finally opened my eyes to the universality of our suffering . . .*

And on and on. Almost every evening, sitting on my porch in the gathering darkness, I would reflect upon the doomed and the spared, the procession of patients with their unfathomable woes flashing before me. In the distance would be the staccato hooting of the red-eyed dove, solitary and cautionary in its plaintive call, reminding me that I was inescapably and, at times, inexplicably in sub-Saharan Africa.

Wikipedia—indeed, my thirty years in medicine—had never prepared me for such things.

# PART 1
# BEGINNINGS

# Chapter 1

# First Rumblings

Although HIV—the human immunodeficiency virus—has been with humans for at least a century, it didn't come to the world's attention until the late 1970s, soon after I had finished medical residency. Thirty years later, at the start of every KITSO course I gave to healthcare workers in Botswana—KITSO was the country's "HIV 101" training, which I headed up—I always told my students how HIV first came to the notice of doctors in America. It was a story most of them had not heard before, but was important for them to know. In the late 1970s, in New York City, Miami, and San Francisco, otherwise healthy young men would crash into hospital emergency rooms with high fevers, hacking cough, and severe shortness of breath, struck down with life-threatening pneumonias. Many of them were so sick that they had to be put on breathing machines in intensive care. Tests showed that they were infected with *Pneumocystis carinii*, an organism that had previously been known to occur only in infants and others with rare cancers. Many patients wouldn't make it despite antibiotic treatment, dying from respiratory failure. At the same time, other patients—again, usually healthy young men—would consult their doctors for odd, purplish spots on their body, often the face and chest. Biopsies would show a previously rare cancer, Kaposi's sarcoma, or KS. The occurrences of this rare pneumonia and cancer flummoxed the specialists, but soon they detected a common thread: most of these men were homosexuals—or else injected drugs intravenously—and they all had a profound lack of an important immune cell, the T-cell, which fights off serious infections. There then quickly followed the identification of the viral culprit and the HIV blood test, as well as, most ominously, shame, guilt, and stigma.

I would tell my KITSO students that at first this immune deficiency disease didn't attract much attention from the public health authorities, for the simple reason of hatred and intolerance: HIV then seemed to infect only gays and drug addicts, "people who didn't matter," as I would put it, gesturing the quotation marks. "As soon as you say certain people 'don't matter' because they're different from you, because you don't approve of them, well, you're on the slippery sliding slope to damnation." Even though many Batswana couldn't conceive of sex between men, let alone shooting up drugs, my KITSO students were much more forgiving than many of us Westerners, and most of them, especially the women, nodded their understanding. The majority of my students, especially the ones who were HIV infected—and there were many of them—already understood the pain of stigma. I would go on to describe the fear—the terror—that Americans felt in the mid-1980s, when they finally realized that this virus was an "equal opportunity pathogen," one that didn't care what sort of sex you were having, or with whom.

Most of my KITSO students were little kids when HIV first hit the headlines in America. At the time, their country had existed as an independent state for only a dozen or so years and seemed the unlikeliest place to be ravaged by HIV. When the first known case of AIDS was reported in Botswana in 1985, the majority of my students were adolescents. At the time, the local authorities—those who even noticed such a thing—assumed that this new disease was, as a doctor friend there once told me, a "gay thing," something that didn't concern them, since, so they reasoned, gay sex was illegal and not practiced in Botswana. It was the same "people who don't matter"—or, in Botswana, people who don't even exist—that had hampered America's early response to the pandemic. Of my more than a few KITSO students who were HIV-infected—a number would come up to me after class and, like penitent to priest, quietly confide that they were positive and were, "thanks be to God," doing well on treatment—many were silently infected during the mid to late 1980s, when HIV was branded a "gay thing."

About the same time that my future students and patients in Africa were being infected, the first reports of a strange immune deficiency disease hit the medical journals in America. I was ensconced in a private medical practice in rural Iowa, far from the outbreak in the big cities. Initially, the journal articles seemed to suggest that the cause was cytomegalovirus, a herpes virus, which somehow destroyed the body's T-cells. There also appeared to be an association with "poppers," the inhaled aphrodisiac used by many gay men—I especially liked this hypothesis, since I never used them. As the body count increased inexorably and the cause was found to be a new virus previously unknown to science, I was both fascinated and terrified. In the sexual revolution of the 1960s and 1970s, before HIV, the worst sexually transmitted disease you could get was herpes, felt to be catastrophic since it messed up your sex life. Now, though, a sexually transmitted virus could kill, usually in ways too terrible to think about. Just as many people go into medicine subconsciously to assuage their fears of death, so I, too, probably got into HIV medicine. Already practicing internal medicine in Iowa, I read all that I could about this new disease. Although the science of HIV was intriguing—a tiny virus targets and kills the body's most crucial immune cells, causing gruesome infections—it was the ethical aspects of this new pandemic that interested me most. Perhaps because I had always felt an outsider, I instinctively reacted with horror at the way people with AIDS were regarded as lepers.

In Iowa, I didn't have any HIV patients, at least not any I knew of. When I moved to West Virginia in the late 1980s, to work at a Veterans Hospital, HIV was still a hypothetical problem—a mysterious disease "out there"—until one evening a medivac helicopter brought in a dying AIDS patient from a small clinic in the boondocks. He was a young guy, a coal miner and former Marine, who had been wasting away in his grandma's trailer in one of the remote, rural "hollers" nestled among the lonely mountains. Someone at the local clinic had sent off an HIV test, and when it came back positive, they immediately shipped him out to us. The doctors and nurses in the emergency room were cocooned in what looked like space suits, protective gear more appropriate for Ebola or chemical weapons. It's anyone's guess what the poor patient thought as the emergency staff gingerly touched him, avoiding as much contact as possible. He was very weak and wasted, and was covered from head to toe with dark-purple blotches of KS. It was a toss-up as to who looked stranger, more extraterrestrial: the disfigured patient or the doctors and nurses in *Star Wars* garb. The poor guy was very short of breath, and was soon gasping for air. In retrospect, he could have had PCP, the "AIDS pneumonia," or even KS pneumonia, but the science of HIV medicine back then was rudimentary. He died less than an hour later, possibly not even knowing he had HIV. The emergency room was decontaminated several times before it was used again. The funeral home back in his small hamlet refused to take the body.

At the same time that we were stressing out in West Virginia over this one AIDS patient—and while my future students and patients in Botswana were unknowingly being infected—the same scenario was being played out in emergency rooms in the big cities on the East and West coasts, only many times a day, day after day, with soul-numbing regularity. And ironically, it was the same sad scenario that I would later witness in Botswana fifteen years later, when people were dying in such numbers that the most thriving businesses in the country were the funeral parlors. But in the gay community in America in the 1980s and 1990s, HIV in Africa wasn't even on the periphery of people's radar screens. I suppose that when you see your friends and loved ones shedding weight, losing their faculties, and eventually dying, your focus becomes constrict, especially if you yourself know you are also infected or fear you might be. The unending procession of obituaries and memorial services for young men previously vibrant and well was an unforgettable legacy of that terrible time. By 1990, countless thousands had died from AIDS in New York City alone.

The stark terror of AIDS in New York was magnified by the guilt and shame attached in those days to homosexuality. Coming down with AIDS meant you were gay—or a drug addict, or both—and stories of guys being abandoned by their families were legion, just as happened in Botswana fifteen years later, when many men would beat up their HIV-infected wives or children and kick them out of home. Early on in America, many people regarded AIDS as a just punishment for people whose sexuality they despised—AIDS sufferers got what they deserved. A prominent conservative magazine pronounced death from AIDS to be "retribution for a repulsive vice." Ironically, the willful indifference of public health officials and politicians helped spread the plague even more. In 1984, several years into the epidemic, New York City had devoted only $24,500 to its AIDS response, and when Congress finally approved funds for AIDS research and education in 1987, it prohibited the use of any money for interventions that "promote, encourage, or condone homosexual activity or the intravenous use of illegal drugs." Discrimination against HIV-infected people was rampant nationwide, in the workplace, at schools, even in the churches. Many hospitals and medical clinics refused to care for them, or else treated them like untouchables, relegated to distant isolation wards. A terrible disease caused by an anonymous virus had been infused with moralism, intolerance, and naked hatred. For many years, the AIDS scene in New York, as well as in the rest of the country, was "a darkling plain swept with confused alarms of struggle and flight, where ignorant armies clash by night."

But there were many heroes during this terrible time, and one of the greatest was Larry Kramer, a gay New Yorker who could never stomach hypocrisy and, when it came to people's lives, stupidity. Calling Kramer an AIDS activist is akin to calling Attila the Hun a wandering traveler. An unrelenting crusader, Kramer was the scourge of politicians, medical authorities, and pharmaceutical companies. Like a wild-eyed biblical prophet crying in the wilderness, he would mercilessly berate the Food and Drug Administration for not moving faster in developing and approving AIDS drugs. By pushing the AIDS treatment agenda forward at a faster pace—his screaming, confrontational style drew media attention as no other person could—Kramer saved tens of thousands of Americans from AIDS. And ironically, by making treatments available sooner and exposing how pharmaceutical companies put profits before lives, Kramer has probably saved more Africans from AIDS than Americans.

When I would tell my KITSO students how HIV first appeared in America, I didn't try to describe any cultural details of the valley of darkness the gay community went through then. The students wouldn't have understood the landscape of gay America, but they definitely understood the fear and shame. Just like New Yorkers in the early 1980s, the Batswana twenty years later were being terrorized by a "mysterious illness." And as with the New York gay community, exceedingly rare was anyone in Botswana who wasn't touched one way or another by the plague stalking the country.

For several years, I watched the unfolding AIDS crisis in New York from the safe remove of Iowa and West Virginia. Geography probably saved me. When I moved to the big city in 1992, to work at an AIDS hospital, I really didn't know what I was getting into. No amount of reading or studying could have prepared me for the alternative universe awaiting me.

# Chapter 2

# In the Thick of It: "The New Face of AIDS"

So much of the story of HIV has been myth and half-truths. In Botswana, AIDS was sometimes regarded as a curse put on you by a powerful witch doctor, which could only be reversed by having sex with a young girl or, worse yet, a baby. In America's AIDS mythology, HIV was widely portrayed for many years—to echo Botswana's initial reaction in the 1980s—as a "gay thing." But statistics have a nasty way of contradicting the common wisdom, and by the late 1980s the CDC, the Centers for Disease Control in the United States, reported that AIDS cases in intravenous (IV) drug users were outpacing those in the gay community. Even more invisible—and reviled—than homosexuals were IV drug addicts, a group that had few advocates, if any. Whereas it might be possible for people to show condescending sympathy for gay men with AIDS—the "love the sinner, hate the sin" cop-out—there was little compassion in 1980s America for people who furtively shot up drugs in back alleys and crack houses, especially when many of them were black and had criminal records.

But by the early 1990s, it was no longer possible to ignore HIV infection in IV drug addicts, or in heterosexuals, women, and people of color, and the media was trumpeting "the new face of AIDS." No one really gave much attention to the pandemic elsewhere in the world, especially in Africa, where the first stream of cases was quietly percolating. HIV is usually a disease in slow motion—it would take five to ten years after infection before the gradual, inexorable decline in T-cells became significant enough to cause AIDS. While "the new face of AIDS" was being heralded in America, my future students and patients in Botswana were already beginning their own slow descent.

My own outlook was likewise constricted, but when I moved to New York City in early 1992 to work at St. Clare's, a decrepit AIDS hospital in Manhattan, I was happy that most of my patients were among the so-called new face of AIDS and not gay white men. As chronicled in my first book, *The Least of These My Brethren*, there were the drug addicts, who would often shoot up—and overdose—in their bathrooms, sometimes using dirty needles they pilfered from the sealed used needles containers in their rooms; the homeless, some of whom would list the bus or train station as their home address, and would bring with them large garbage bags or even shopping carts full of their possessions; the prisoners and ex-prisoners, many of whom would claim they got HIV from "dirty women," and not from their "bitches" in prison, or from shooting up drugs; the mentally ill, whose antics would sometimes drive us doctors crazy, especially when they had drug-resistant TB and wouldn't stay in their isolation rooms, or would abscond altogether; the criminals, who would flagrantly have sex with their girlfriends in front of their roommates or would insist on smoking next to their oxygen tanks; the transvestites, who, decked out with make-up lovingly applied at their bedside by their "sister" drag queens, would look absolutely fabulous as they breathed their last; and anyone else who lacked insurance—including a few gay white males—or who would definitely seem out of place at the city's renowned medical centers. Many patients had the triple whammy of HIV dementia, active drug use, and major personality disorders. Too often "the new face of AIDS" was not very pretty, its sufferers not very heroic or easily evoking sympathy.

St. Clare's was an alternative universe, full of misfits—and that was just among its medical staff. Anonymously tucked away in unsavory low-rise tenement buildings in Hell's Kitchen, it was really the largest Designated AIDS Center in the state, although shabby and worn down with a bad case of the 1950s. The Catholic Church owned the place—a large picture of His Eminence, John Cardinal O'Connor, in full scarlet regalia greeted visitors at the entrance, and innumerable crucifixes and statues of the Blessed Virgin adorned rooms and hallways. And there were the usual Catholic strictures against condoms and discussion of safe sex, which everyone ignored, especially the pastoral care staff. Father Jack, the renegade, world-weary priest for the hospital, reveled in the letters of reprimand from his Monsignor—a particularly contentious one was "four pages long, *single-spaced!*"—and he once quipped that "all the Church cares about is tits and dicks!" The medical staff was equally color-ful, with revolutionaries, sex fiends, manic-depressives, and other-wise odd personalities that perfectly melded with the craziness of the patients.

I was at St. Clare's when there were no effective treatments for HIV. We would give AZT, but its side effects often made patients sicker and it usually didn't work anyway. Our patients were incred-ibly sick, dim shadows of their former selves, many with T-cell counts of zero—the normal count should be over five hundred. True, we could often treat the severe infections they'd come in with, even sending them home after they recovered. But they always bounced back, eventually for the last time. Fifteen years later in Bot-swana, when life-saving HIV drugs were finally available, the situa-tion was perversely reversed: when AIDS patients were hospitalized with the same life-threatening infections my St. Clare's patients had had, there was actually hope, *if* we could get them over their acute

AIDS-related problems, so they could then start the HIV drugs. But as dysfunctional as St. Clare's was, it was the Mayo Clinic compared with hospitals in Botswana, where many patients would slip through our fingers and into the grave, losing their chance for HIV treatment.

At St. Clare's, we tried not only to help patients recover from their acute AIDS infections, but also to help them put things right in their lives, to get beyond the abuse, pain, and loneliness that had characterized their broken lives for so many years before they were struck down with AIDS. These were patients whom most people on the outside had always ignored, avoided, or treated with contempt. I liked to hope that for some of our patients we gave them precious time before they died to set things right with their families and friends and, above all, with themselves, but we'll never know. A kind gesture to a patient wasting away to nothing, patience for a withdrawing crack-head, words of reassurance to mothers grieving the loss of their sons—these were as important as properly dosing antibiotics for their serious infections.

St. Clare's was the first time I came up against the full horror of AIDS. Never before had I cared for so many patients so far gone, never before had I seen so much death face to face. Helping me—and countless patients—deal with such suffering was Sister Pascal Conforti, St. Clare's director of pastoral care, who, with understated compassion and singular strength of spirit, was always there to ease the lonely anguish of so many of our patients. Avoiding any overt religiosity—the small crucifix around her neck was the only clue she was a nun—she reassured patients that is was OK to let go, "to go to a far better place." I came to rely on her to ease the pain that morphine could not touch, to give solace to the despair that Prozac could not reach, to understand the "difficult" patient that psychiatry could not fathom. Quietly observing patients' suffering with mindfulness and grace, Pascal was St. Clare's sentinel presence, its guardian angel.

My AIDS ward was a crucible of despair and hope, and it taught me many lessons, perhaps the greatest of which is that *we are all HIV-positive in this weary sojourn called life*. The distinction between the HIV-infected and the HIV-uninfected is illusory, since suffering and death are our universal destinies. This realization could neutralize the shame and stigma the virus had engendered. Before Botswana, I always used to say that St. Clare's was the best job I'd ever had, crystallizing my commitment to caring for "the other," the many marginalized people with AIDS.

Today, St. Clare's Hospital is no more, a victim of medical science's battle against HIV. At the Vancouver AIDS Conference in 1996, the first life-saving HIV treatments were announced to frenzied applause. The new ARVs—antiretroviral drugs, which short-circuit the virus and keep it from multiplying—gave the body's decimated immune system a chance to repair itself. Patients were literally getting out of their deathbeds, returning to their former selves. Even minds ravaged by HIV dementia were gradually restored. As AIDS patients were no longer coming into the hospital, St. Clare's patient census was dropping and, with it, the money the state was paying for their care. As I would rhapsodically tell my KITSO students ten years later in Botswana, whole hospital wards were shut down across the city, and medical staff were let go. Nowadays, walking past the renovated luxury tenements that once housed this remarkable sanctuary for the forlorn and forgotten, you wouldn't even know that a hospital had once been there.

# Chapter 3

# First Forays into Africa

By 1992, epidemiologists were saying that Africa was irretrievably lost to HIV/AIDS, with less hope than we had in the States. Back then, when we were caught up in the HIV outbreak in America, Africa was the silent, smoldering center of the epidemic, which was silently spreading through its villages and cities with alarming speed. The statistics were sobering: the World Health Organization (WHO) estimated that the number of HIV-infected Africans had increased from 2.5 million in 1987 to five million in 1995. By 1992, the year I started at St. Clare's, it was estimated that 20 percent of young adults in Botswana were infected, some of them the doctors and nurses I would later teach HIV medicine. In Francistown, Botswana's second-largest city, nearly half of all pregnant women showing up at the main hospital were positive for HIV, risking transmission of the virus to their babies. Because HIV was a disease in slow motion, the initial numbers of AIDS cases in Africa were only a few hundred in the early 1990s, but the trickle soon became a torrent—a tsunami—that threatened to reverse the major gains African countries had made against TB, malaria, and other diseases.

The lack of any HIV treatments was one thing—they wouldn't appear until 1996 in the States—but most African countries didn't even have the antibiotics and trained healthcare workers to treat patients' opportunistic infections. Buying time, keeping AIDS patients alive until HIV drugs were developed, wasn't an option in Africa. The projection of millions upon millions of Africans dying from AIDS—including babies and children—was mind-numbing.

In late 1992, still a newbie at St. Clare's, I went to Cameroon, for the 7th International AIDS in Africa Conference, more as a lark than anything else. Cameroon's dense tropical forests were probably where HIV jumped from chimpanzees to man over a century ago. From the moment my plane landed in Duala, the post-apocalyptic slum on the Gulf of Guinea, I realized I was in a completely different world. The tropical humidity condensing on the airplane's windows obscured any view of the dilapidated terminal. In customs, a "helpful" bystander, undoubtedly in on the scam, advised me to bribe "the captain" there so I could avoid any delay. Half-crazed from jet lag, I think I gave him five hundred francs, and the "captain" absent-mindedly passed his hands over my luggage, looking up blankly at the ceiling. I had originally planned to make the three-hour bus ride from Duala to Yaounde, the capital and conference venue, but when I asked conference staff greeting us at the airport if the bus was safe, their cheerful reply, uttered without sarcasm or satire, was "It's safe as long as there are no armed attacks!" Because there was a rebel insurgency in the remote parts of the country, I opted for an Air Cameroon flight later in the day.

But as I quickly learned, things in Africa were seldom easy. Although I was at the front of the ticket counter at the Air Cameroon office, it took almost three hours to buy the ticket to Yaounde—the computer was up and down, and other customers would push in front of me, the ticket agent breaking away to help them while I tried to stay calm. The flight to Yaoundé later that afternoon was overbooked beyond belief, giving a whole new meaning to "open seating," as what seemed like thousands of us frantically ran with our luggage to board the very old 737. Outpacing the elderly and infirm, I collapsed into a tattered aisle seat. There was a delay in departure, because the flight attendants couldn't close the front door. Finally—I saw it all from my seat—one of the male attendants executed an impressive kick-jump and slammed the sucker shut.

At the entrance to my hotel in Yaoundé, soldiers lazed about in their jeeps, sub-machine guns idly dangling by their sides. Night and day, the hotel's corridors were trolled by young women, ostensibly conference staff, but their penetrating glances indicated they weren't there to provide guidance on the local tour sites.

The conference was held atop one of the city's hills, at an immense hall built by the Cubans years earlier and falling into disrepair. Most of the attendees were Africans, with a smattering of Europeans and the odd American or two. The head of WHO was supposed to attend but backed out at the last minute. Since it was 1992 and no HIV treatments were on the horizon, almost all of the lectures and sessions were about safe sex and bare-bones medical care—aspirin, morphine, salves—usually provided by nurses and volunteer workers going from village to village. Unlike medical conferences in the States, no major pharmaceutical companies attended with their flashy booths and free trinkets. Also absent were any "names" in HIV medicine from the States—Africa just wasn't on their agendas then. There were only a few sessions on clinical research in Africa, but there were plenty of presentations about the bleak epidemiology of the pandemic there.

One afternoon, I joined some French doctors at the conference for a walk around the bustling market in the downtown, and we struck up conversations with several vendors, who easily identified us as conference attendees. As if to prove a point to himself, one of them challenged us over whether HIV was a problem he needed to worry about: "Look at me: I've had sex with hundreds of women, and I feel totally fine! This HIV is not true! Not true!" People around him nodded their support, some of them laughing at our seeming cluelessness. We were dumbfounded, but couldn't rebut the man's tirade. I've often wondered whether he is still alive.

Cameroon was my first foray into Africa, and I lived not only to tell about it but also to wonder whether I could work there. But once safely back in New York, I quickly became engulfed in the day-to-day demands of St. Clare's, as well as in acclimatizing to my new life in the city. Besides, without any life-saving HIV treatments available even in the States, Africa would have to wait.

＿＿＿

After ignoring HIV in the late 1980s and early 1990s, America started pouring tens of millions into treating the country's former lepers. Public health authorities finally realized that HIV wasn't just a "gay thing," and that it needed serious attention, lest it spread to respectable middle-class heterosexuals. Once HIV patients started ARVs and stopped dying, money for treating them poured in. By the late 1990s in America, HIV was a major cottage industry in the health care system, spawning tens of thousands of jobs. Administrators, bureaucrats, medical directors, program directors, counselors, social workers—the list seemed endless—had good jobs flowing directly from HIV money. Since there was no talk of a "cure" and ARV treatment was lifelong, your job was secure.

In the late 1990s, I became medical director of the Ryan Center, a large community health center in Manhattan, which chiefly cared for the poor, including a large number of HIV patients, most doing well on the new treatments. At Ryan, I witnessed first-hand the AIDS bureaucracy that thrived on "HIV exceptionalism," the belief that, because of its stigma, HIV had to be regarded as a unique, special condition. Thanks to heavy lobbying by the advocates, HIV patients in New York State were the recipients of major benefits not available to non-HIV patients: housing, food stamps, free medical care, free medications, free transportation to the clinic, intensive social work assistance, and comprehensive mental health care. There were even stories of some HIV-negative people becoming infected intentionally, so they could enjoy such benefits. Later in Botswana, my HIV patients had nothing in the way of social service support, no army of social workers, counselors, or mental health staff to help them. The most they got was a monthly "food basket" with canned goods, rice, flour, and some vegetables, which would last them a week or so. And even then, many of the nurses, skeptical and reproving, would give them the third degree to find out whether they really needed assistance or were just malingering.

So in New York State, HIV patients were highly valuable commodities: diagnosing a new HIV patient was akin to finding a gold nugget. So prized were such patients that hospitals and clinics routinely tried to steal them from one another. The money to care for these patients was granted by government bureaucrats whom we treated like major potentates to be courted and sucked up to. It was all pretty unseemly, but I found myself up to my neck in it. Although we all acted as if we were doing God's work, none of us were saints, or even close to it.

———————

After three years at Ryan, I had had enough of American health care—HIV was well under control, with newer and newer ARVs on the market, with fewer and fewer side effects—and I eagerly attended the International AIDS Conference in Durban, South Africa, along with my best friend. It was the first major AIDS conference held in a developing country. After being ignored, Africans were now drawing major attention, if only out of guilt at our having so much and their having nothing. Furthermore, like sharks smelling fresh blood in the water, the drug companies sensed a vast, untouched market for their ARV's, now that there was serious discussion in the West about funneling billions of dollars for HIV treatment into Africa. Although altruism did play a role in America's international HIV initiatives, there was also serious worry that AIDS might destabilize the few democracies in Africa, Botswana and South Africa among them. Both of these countries were projected to suffer death on an unimaginable scale.

As opposed to the Cameroon meeting eight years earlier, the Durban conference was teeming with all of the world's major HIV players—UNAIDS, the WHO, the CDC, major medical centers in Europe and the States, big-time researchers, major pharmaceutical companies, human rights organizations, wild-eyed advocates, government leaders, and politicians. Celebrities mingled with multibillionaire philanthropists, all under the glare of worldwide media. Also among the throngs clogging the hallways of the conference center were more than a few entrepreneurs, wheeler-dealers who, like the drug companies, felt there was substantial money to be made in AIDS and were positioning themselves to get grants from donor countries. Although most of these grant dollars would go to AIDS care, the fees they could skim off for administrative costs, including their own generous salaries, were substantial.

Durban in 2000 was where science collided with ignorance and denialism: South Africa's President Thabo Mbeki, who was educated enough to know better, was booed when he spouted the nonsense that HIV didn't cause AIDS. A few weeks before the conference, over five thousand doctors and researchers signed the Durban Declaration, attesting rather obviously that HIV was the cause of AIDS. At that point in the epidemic, it was like proclaiming that the earth was round, not flat. The Mbeki government pressured South African scientists not to sign it, saying it was "elitist" and belonged in the "dustbin." His Minister of Health, Dr. Tshabalala-Msimang, dubbed "Dr. Beetroot," claimed that beets, garlic, and other vegetables, not the ARVs of the West, would reverse the immune deficiency. Later studies would show that Mbeki's willful ignorance and intellectual conceit probably cost the lives of at least 300,000 South Africans. Many of the westerners attending Durban, most of whom were white, felt awkward about this debate, since they didn't want to appear racist or "politically incorrect" in telling an African leader he was out of his mind. Nelson Mandela, the former President, closed the conference with a lackluster speech. Everyone had hoped for a more robust rebuttal of AIDS denialism, but then again, he was frail and didn't want to confront his successor directly. Besides, he had already done enough for his country: he had set them free to make their own mistakes, and hopefully to learn from them.

Right after the conference, before leaving for the States, my friend and I took a half-day private tour of Johannesburg, which is just a few hundred miles from Botswana. Like the rest of the country, the city seemed both African and European. The once prosperous downtown was rundown and seedy, but bustling with black Africans going about their business. Former high-rise luxury hotels and once beautiful Art Deco apartment buildings, previously the preserve of privileged whites, were now gutted and dilapidated, jam-packed with squatters and drug dealers, although many buildings had no electricity because the copper wiring had been ripped out years earlier. When Apartheid ended, fearful whites emptied out the city core and fled to the suburbs, where gated communities were surrounded by high walls mounted with razor-sharp barbed wire and security alarms.

That afternoon, before our late-evening flight out, we visited Soweto, the vast township outside the city and home to over a million people. True, there were endless shacks packed tightly together and stretching far beyond the horizon, but there were also middle-class areas as well. Out driver took us to the Mandela House, a touristy stop which was one of Mandela's homes after he was released from prison. At the house's gift shop at the end of tour, as we were signing the visitor register, my friend, who was well-meaning but also had a big mouth, told the two young women there that we had been at the Durban conference and that I was an "AIDS doctor."

Both of them immediately surrounded me, shook my hands, and exclaimed repeatedly, "God bless you, doctor! Please stay and help us!" The earnestness—desperation—of their praises and entreaties was too much to bear, and we quickly retreated to our waiting car.

Later that night, as our Sabena Airlines jumbo-jet lifted off from Johannesburg International into the darkness, I looked down on the city's lights and thought about the two women at the Mandela House. I wondered whether I would someday return to treat AIDS patients in Africa.

The Durban conference finally planted the seed, and in 2001, less than a year later, I finally came face-to-face with the *real* "new face of AIDS," the face of AIDS in Africa. It was an experience forever seared in my memory.

I was in Kampala, Uganda, interviewing for a job with an American university that had a research outpost there. One morning I went on rounds with one of the teams of medical residents at Mulago Hospital, the medical school's teaching hospital and the largest in Uganda. At the entrance to the hospital was a herd of cows, contentedly resting under the trees. Waiting for visiting hours, scores of family members, many with bags of food and small washbasins for bathing their loved ones, were lounging under the covered walkways connecting the one-story hospital wards. Goats frolicked between the wards, helping themselves to the trash bins. At the time, I was jet-lagged and overwhelmed by the strangeness of the country, and I really cannot remember much more from that morning, save for one of the patients we saw on our rounds, a young woman with AIDS and TB. Admitted to the male medical ward—the female ward was packed full—she was in a bed off to the side, an ancient privacy screen affording only perfunctory seclusion.

Very wasted, practically skeletal, she struggled to sit up as we approached her bed, finally propping herself halfway up with an outstretched arm behind her. She had prominent ribs, shrunken sagging breasts, practically no muscle mass. Her open tattered sundress hung loosely on her wisp of a body. She was a starkly eloquent image of AIDS in Africa. Almost ten years earlier, at St. Clare's, I had seen similarly dire patients many times, years before life-saving treatments came on the scene. But I had never seen a gaze like hers, emanating deep from her sunken bony orbits. Sure, many such stares were due to HIV dementia rotting the brain, but this woman's eyes seemed to evince profound awareness of her extremity, of her impending mortality. A prolonged coughing jag interrupted her meditation, and she struggled to find something into which she could spit her blood-streaked phlegm, finally using her brightly colored scarf, which, except for a worn Bible beside her pillow, appeared to be the only personal possession she had.

Who was she? Definitely someone's daughter, once young and filled with the hopes of childhood. Perhaps someone's partner, mother, aunt, or sister. Later on, when I was fully immersed in AIDS in Botswana, I would realize that many of her family—parents, children, partner, siblings—might well have gone before her, victims of the same contagions now rattling her body. How did she get to this penultimate way station? And what, or who, was she thinking about? Most likely, she didn't even know that in better-resourced countries she could have received ARVs that might have nursed her back to health. Although HIV medicines were undoubtedly available somewhere in Kampala, they were light years beyond her meagre means, since Uganda had no HIV treatment program at the time.

This woman was my first African AIDS patient. But within a few years, such patients would be legion for me. At that moment, I was determined more than ever to become an AIDS doctor in Africa. Six months later, I would receive the momentous telephone call about a job in Botswana, a call that would ultimately transform me in ways I had never imagined.

# PART 2

# THE GREAT EXPERIMENT BEGINS: BOTSWANA 2002–2008

# Chapter 4

# Not a Community of Mother Teresa's

What is now Botswana had been in territorial limbo for centuries, quietly wedged among German, Dutch, and English colonies. Mostly arid bush, the region hadn't been of interest to anyone until the late nineteenth century, when Dutch Boers to the south started making incursions into the area. The popular mythology has it that about this time "the three chiefs" from the major tribes there journeyed to London, to petition Queen Victoria for protection. In a memorial in the center of Gaborone, Botswana's eventual capital, are three larger-than-life statues of the chiefs, solemn and distinguished in their Victorian suits. In fact, as part of the infamous scramble for Africa, Great Britain had already decided to take over the area—it was really more of an afterthought than anything else—and in 1885 the Protectorate of Bechuanaland stumbled into being.

Largely ignored throughout the first half of the twentieth century, Bechuanaland stoically muddled along, never attaining the dignity of colony status like its much larger neighbor South Africa. But by the 1960s, having long passed its colonial zenith, Britain was running out of money and decided to unload large parts of its costly empire, including its sleepy little protectorate in southern Africa. The tribal leaders in Bechuanaland really weren't keen for independence—as colonizers, the Brits were pretty benign—but the locals had no choice. Britain's infamous "golden handshake" for territories it no longer wanted—a gift of gold bullion—sealed the deal, and independence was granted in 1966. A bit embarrassed by how little they had done for the country—they really hadn't given it any significant infrastructure up to that point—the British left behind a few paltry government buildings, a paved road, and a new hospital, Princess Marina, which 40 years later became known as a place where people went to die from AIDS. Marina was named after the Greek princess who had married into the British royal family earlier in the century. She represented the Crown at the formal independence celebrations in 1966—apparently Elizabeth II couldn't have been bothered to attend herself. Such had been the fate of Botswana, taken for granted, never really on anyone's radar screen. But the country had a last laugh of sorts on the Brits: soon after independence, diamonds were discovered—in seemingly endless supply—and then uranium, and then platinum, and nickel, and enough coal to power all of Africa for centuries to come. It was one of God's many little jokes involving this small, beleaguered country.

I really had no idea what I was getting myself into when I accepted the job in Botswana. When the British Airways 747 touched down in Johannesburg in September 2002, I had a mini panic attack over what I had just done: I'd left friends and family—to say nothing about my dear dog—as well as a high-profile, high-paying job for a vague position in a country I knew next to nothing about. Then again, I was seriously jet-lagged and hung over from too much wine and green Sambuca the night before on my stopover in Rome. I somehow managed to catch my flight to Gaborone later that morning. As the small Air Botswana airplane banked and made its final approach into the Sir Seretse Khama International Airport a few miles outside the capital, I peered down at the ground and saw only flat squat bush, with a few isolated huts and houses surrounded by arid ground, as well as what I later learned were warthogs darting in and out of the vegetation. No lush green tropical forests as in Cameroon or rolling hills of rich farmland as in South Africa. Pretty dull and boring. Welcome to Botswana.

I had come to Botswana to work for ACHAP, the African Comprehensive HIV/AIDS Partnerships, the remarkable collaboration that the Bill and Melinda Gates Foundation and Merck Pharmaceuticals had entered into with the government of Botswana. By the late 1990s, it was finally apparent to the government that HIV was not a "gay thing," and that this largely unheralded country was doomed to near-extinction if something decisive wasn't done, and done quickly. Probably responsible for saving well over 100,000 of his countrymen—he really deserved a Nobel Prize—President Festus Mogae, a jovial and portly politician of the ruling Botswana Democratic Party, had the foresight and courage to accept offers of help from Bill Gates and Merck. Mogae, who had been Oxford-educated, was intended by the political elite to only be a place-holder, a competent Chief Executive until "the boy," Ian Khama, son of the nation's founding President, Sir Seretse Khama, was mature enough to become President in his own right. Like his father, Ian was royalty, with a lineage going back several centuries. After college in the UK, he headed up the Botswana Defense Force, the country's army, which had always been his first love, and in 1998 he became vice-president under Mogae.

So, in the late 1990s President Mogae decided that something had to be done about HIV in his country. At that time it really wasn't clear whether offers of help from the West would even make a difference, but he took a leap of faith. Merck agreed to provide the ARVs free of charge, and Gates provided the money to bring over people like me to help with the start-up of treatment. If Mogae had not been President back then, the history of Botswana's HIV crisis might have been very different.

Botswana's HIV/AIDS Treatment Programme had started up, haltingly and glacially, several months before my arrival in late 2002. It was the very first one on the continent, an experiment which everyone was watching closely to see if it would work, if Africans could muster the resources to snatch people from the grave. As I would soon observe, it was a very messy and haphazard process—an entire country was turned inside out and upside down in the most profound ways.

By the time I arrived, Botswana was teeming with outsiders, largely Westerners who were ostensibly there to help its fledgling Treatment Programme. As the weeks wore on, the full scope of the unfolding chaos and complexity of the Treatment Programme became apparent. It was akin to a raucous gold-mining town in the wild and woolly west, only here, instead of gold, many of the outsiders were angling for lucrative consultancies or ground-breaking medical research, mining for clinical data to add luster to their CVs. Some of them were there simply for the adventure, including trips to see wild animals in the many game reserves up north. I thought I was there to help people with AIDS, but as I would soon find out, to my great sorrow, it wasn't so simple.

There were lots of characters there. A colleague of mine at ACHAP, an internist from India, once loudly proclaimed, "There's money to be made from AIDS, and I intend to have some of it!" She was the same person who held forth that all marital relationships should be on five-year contracts, with the option to move on after that.

One of the major players when I arrived was a young American doctor who never did his residency after medical school and instead had joined a high-powered international consultancy, a job which he was soon able to segue into a powerful position in the Treatment Programme. He was like an AIDS tsar, liaising between ACHAP and the government. He was very bright and a facile speaker, but after his lengthy disquisitions, jam-packed with jargon like "stakeholders" and "terms of reference," I never could completely figure out exactly what he had said. After a few years, he left Botswana and started up his own health care consultancy in South Africa. Its website is quite impressive, and highlights his role in the start-up of Botswana's Treatment Programme. Those of us who were actually there, on the ground, seeing patients and dealing with the Programme close-up, have a somewhat different take on the matter. There were lots of people who saw opportunity amid the AIDS crisis. It was definitely not a religious community of Mother Teresa's. But then again, you don't have to be a saint to save someone from AIDS.

Although there were always entrepreneurs circling around the National Treatment Programme, there were also good people from the West. If it weren't for "Bible Bill" Wester and Hermann Bussmann, doctors from Harvard and truly nice guys, the Treatment Programme wouldn't have started when it did in early 2002. The government was then frozen in characteristic "I've-fallen-and-can't-get-up" mode—the numerous byzantine committees and agencies were too hamstrung by bureaucratic inertia to actually start treating patients. Bill and Hermann, with crucial help from their Batswana nursing staff, just started treating patients. And so Marina Hospital's HIV clinic, the first in the nation, lurched into being. True, as with many of us, their reasons were complex: they needed the Treatment Programme to start before they could undertake a big clinical research study for Harvard. But they probably would have done it anyway. And oddly enough, they didn't later parlay their experience into a moneymaking consultancy.

Arriving back in their home country right as the Treatment Programme started were two truly remarkable heroes, Dr. Ndwapi Ndwapi and Dr. Tendani Gaolathe, the co-directors of the Marina Hospital AIDS clinic. When I first met them, they were in their early thirties and were the future of medicine in Botswana. After secondary education in Botswana, they had gone to college together in America, followed by medical school and residency there. Even if she had not been the daughter of an important government minister, Tendani would still have been fearlessly outspoken on behalf of her fellow citizens with AIDS, with a steely resolve. Six months after Marina's AIDS clinic had opened in 2002, Kofi Annan, Secretary General of the United Nations, visited the clinic, escorted by the senior physician in the Ministry of Health. It had not been lost on Tendani that this was the first visit to the country's first AIDS clinic by any high-ranking official from the ministry. As soon as the doctor from the ministry introduced Tendani to Mr. Annan, she replied pointedly to the bureaucrat, in front of the Secretary General, "Well, doctor, I see it took Kofi Annan to get you to finally visit us here." The guy just squirmed and smiled.

Like Tendani, Ndwapi also showed a wealth of wisdom and insight, probably from working as a youth in the political campaigns of his father, who had been a member of parliament for many years. Less than a year into the Treatment Programme, he was summoned to BOTUSA to answer questions from some CDC people who were in town. BOTUSA was the collaboration between the Botswana government and the US Centers for Disease Control and Prevention, and was heavily involved in doling out money for the Treatment Programme. "It was the same old question about how many people we have on treatment so far," Ndwapi told me afterwards. "I told them we don't have reliable numbers yet, that it's still too early, but they still wanted a number. So I turned to them and said, 'Tell me: how many people does the United States have on treatment?' That shut them up." Aware that no one at the CDC could quote the number of Americans on ARV therapy—and effective HIV treatments had been on the scene in the States for over seven years at the time—Ndwapi always had a disarming way of highlighting double standards.

After completing their medical residencies in America, Ndwapi and Tendani returned to Botswana to help with the AIDS crisis, drawing subsistence-level government salaries. When early on

I praised Ndwapi for returning, and not staying in America for a six-figure income, he replied, with characteristic directness, "Dr. Baxter, it never once occurred to me not to return to Botswana." These two doctors were the real story behind Botswana's HIV/AIDS Treatment Programme, as they worked tirelessly for many years in Marina's AIDS clinic. Whenever I was interviewed by science writers and reporters briefly visiting to write about this great experiment, I always urged them to interview Ndwapi and Tendani, but they never did.

A big problem during these early years was that no one really knew who was in charge. No one was, but everyone was. As a result, nobody was willing to make any decisions. I once saw a diagram of the many government agencies and committees involved in the Treatment Programme, the type with arrows and lines connecting the individual fiefdoms of government, all ultimately leading up to the Office of the President. Its arcane complexity was a tribute to the bureaucratic mind. During one of the early years of the Treatment Programme, the Ministry of Health, hamstrung by its own bureaucracy, had to return 70 million pula to the government unspent—at the time, ten million dollars, enough to fund a dozen new HIV clinics in the country. The Batswana's penchant for obtuse bureaucracy and overelaborate governmental rituals had been inherited from the Brits. They wanted to be led by a Prince Charles, when what they really needed was Arnold Schwarzenegger's Terminator.

During my first months in Gaborone, I kept largely to myself, and in the evenings retreated to my bedroom, listening to music and reading. Although I had a nice three-bedroom house entirely to myself, I basically lived in my bedroom, detached and aloof. In the clinics, I impassively observed my patients' suffering, pronounced their lives to be as important as—no, *more* important—than those of people in the States, and then retired to my bedroom, to Bach and Mozart, maybe even to write a book about my stay. My grandiosity was the purity of my mission there, as well as my increasing contempt for the whining, demanding, entitled patients in America. I really had nothing of substance to learn, especially about myself. Nothing, that is, until I crashed into the harsh realities of AIDS in Africa, with catastrophic results for two Batswana, Comfort and Polite—actually three, if you count Polite's baby boy.

# Chapter 5

## Crash and Burn

Comfort spent all of her ten years of life in Old Naledi, Gaborone's slum and oldest neighborhood. Tourists, on break from safaris up north, would often photograph its bleak shacks from the safe remove of the adjacent road, to document for folks back home that they had witnessed African poverty. Over the decades, factories had sprouted up haphazardly next to the community, some of them dumping toxic waste into nearby ditches. Many of its residents worked at these businesses, usually at the minimum wage of six hundred pula a month, or approximately 125 dollars.

Most of Old Naledi's houses were very old, dating from before independence in 1966, when Gaborone was a small village with one dirt road. The one-room dwellings, all mud or brick, were tightly packed together, their sheet-metal roofs anchored by large rocks for summer's windstorms. Some of the houses had small yards, bare and treeless and without the high walls and security fences in more upscale areas of the capital. Old Naledi's narrow dirt streets were potholed and rutted, largely populated by playing children, as well as the ubiquitous chickens, goats, and scrawny dogs. The only color to the place was given by the clothes hung out to dry in the yards. Most of the abodes had no indoor plumbing, and outhouses—"long drops"—abutted against the houses. Water had to be carried from the half-dozen or so taps scattered throughout the community. Hidden in the backyards and narrow spaces were illegal home-made alcohol stills to relieve the monotony. Old Naledi's poverty was not as stark or dangerous as that of the awesome shantytowns of neighboring South Africa or the densely packed slums of Zambia's capital, Lusaka. It was relatively safe during the day, but visits there at night could be dicey. Every month or so, at payday, a worker returning home to Old Naledi would be robbed of her month's wages.

Soon after my arrival in Botswana, I met Aaron, a white African of Jewish descent who had moved from Zimbabwe to Gaborone a few years earlier with his wife and children—his family farm of four generations had been confiscated by President Mugabe's henchmen. He owned a landscaping and brush-clearing company, headquartered not far from Old Naledi. Most of his several dozen employees lived in Old Naledi. Daily they would be ferried to work sites throughout the city, where they would clear brush, trim trees, and tend the verdant yards and gardens of the well-to-do. Tall and drop-dead handsome, he was a good boss, paying them a few hundred pula above the minimum wage, even when prolonged rainstorms made it impossible to work.

Soon after we met, Aaron recounted the sad, recurring story played out every day throughout the country at businesses such as his, especially ones with minimum-wage employees. A worker would gradually start losing weight, slowly becoming weaker and weaker. Bosses and co-workers, much as New Yorkers did in the 1980s and 1990s, would pretend not to notice, averting their eyes from the marked person. Then came frequent missed days at work. A few months later, after a prolonged absence from the job, word would seep through that the employee had returned to their family in their home village. Soon thereafter news would arrive of the worker's death. No one ever asked the cause of death, and no one wanted to know, even though most of the time the person had been young and once vibrant.

The following weekend, the deceased's co-workers would pile into a kombi, a large van, to attend their friend's funeral, which, as was the custom, would almost always be an elaborate affair, with an abundance of prepared food and not inconsiderable drink. Families were expected to put on a good show, even if it impoverished them further. At all such funerals, the cause of death would never be discussed—to name it was taboo—but the specter of a capricious foe always lurked in the background. Months later, the cycle would repeat itself, with the same predictable outcome, as yet another worker succumbed to the same mysterious illness.

Minimum-wage workers such as Aaron's had no medical insurance, and relied on care at government clinics. Largely superstitious and fearful of AIDS, they knew little, if anything, about how to access Botswana's nascent National ARV Programme, let alone how to get HIV tested. Terrified of HIV's seemingly inevitable visitation, they seemed resigned to be at its whim, like prey to the predator.

A few weeks after we had met, Aaron asked me to stop by his business, to talk to his staff about HIV prevention and treatment. *"Tell them there'll be no more dying!"* he thundered, with almost apostolic fervor.

A few days later, close to knocking-off time, I showed up at Aaron's company. The workers, all young women dressed in dark-blue jumpsuits, crowded around me. The job foreman acted as translator, but most of the employees understood some English—universal education in Botswana had touched even the poorest citizens.

"There should be no more dying from AIDS," I declared, trying my best to mimic my friend. "AIDS in Botswana no longer means death!" The workers smiled and listened attentively. A visit from a doctor was a new thing for them, and it at least broke the monotony of an otherwise routine day. I told them that, as citizens, they were entitled to free care if they came down with AIDS. I handed out government brochures about HIV, printed in both English and Setswana. But the real treats were the colored enamel AIDS pins, which they proudly affixed to their uniforms. I also handed out my card, with my mobile phone number, in case they had any questions or needed medical help. "Just call and hang up and I'll call you back." I knew that even the briefest local phone call was too expensive for them.

As expected, there were no questions, but the workers probably understood what I was on about. Even this early into the National Programme, Botswana was awash with AIDS-prevention messages, from the radio and TV, newspaper advertisements, and billboards screaming out that AIDS kills and that abstinence, monogamy, and condoms would save the day. As I left, I was showered with merry shouts, "Our doctor! Our doctor!"

Thereafter, on a weekly basis, I visited Aaron's company, both to hang out with my new friend and to remind his workers that I was available to help them. They were always happy to see me, and always insisted on hand-washing my car. Effusively shouting "Our doctor! Our doctor!" they seemed full of life, and not the fatalistic prey Aaron had spoken of. But no one yet ventured to step forward to ask for help. A month or so after I started my visits, one of the workers, Mpho, who was shyer and quieter than the others, took me aside and gave me a story she had written by hand on lined essay paper. She asked if I could get it published in an AIDS brochure, like the ones I had given out on my first visit:

*SUGA DADDY (MONEY MONSTER)*

*One day, walking from school facing down, I heard a hooter, I raise my head.*
*Near my feet, there was a nice car, jaguar, a portable car indeed.*

*A man in his fifty's smiles and waves his hand to me.*
*'Babe,' please come to me. Want a lift?*
*'Come on, don't disappoint me, I can give you everything,*
  *everything you want please.'*

*He opened the door for me.*
*'Come on have a seat.' We drive away.*
*'Let's get something to eat.'*

*He drive to the Nando's restaurant.*
*He buy two boxes of Nando's and soft drinks.*
*'Let's start eating.' I was so scared.*
*'Come on, don't be a fool.'*
*I force myself to eat because I can't take them home because my*
  *mom would like to know and cut off my head.*

*He promise me many many things.*
*Trip to Sun City, but never come.*
*He gave me p100 for lunch.*
*Oh tomorrow 'Babe' at our stop.*
*This will take away your sorrow.*

*Tomorrow comes. He was the first one at our stop.*
*He drive to the nearby bush.*
*There he park.*
*He touch my small back with his big hand. Hot sweat running*
  *on my back. I push it away. Please, 'Babe', I can't 'kill' you.*
  *Trust me, please.*

*Things fall apart. Sex without a condom.*
*Things keep on changing. My studies and responsibilities forgot.*
*A new life growing inside me.*

*Monthly period never*
*come. I was 'pregnant'!*
*I told sugar daddy. He said 'What? Mma, I'm married, legally*
    *married. Out, out of my car and set me free! What a fool!'*

*Everything was dark for I could only mourn my babe, my school*
    *and my life.*
*I go for blood test with my mom. Then the results 'RED MARK!'*
    *HIV-positive.*
*Every thread of my future is torn.*
*HIV 'AIDS' has stolen my life.*
*Girls take care, don't follow my footsteps.*
*Why should we die rather than changing.*

*People, why don't we take action.*
*Why don't we change our mind.*
*Why don't we change our behaviour.*

*Batswana 'Betsho', why we let our kids to be orphans.*
*Why don't we change our attitude.*
*Why we let HIV 'AIDS' to ruin our lives.*

*People knows all over but we don't change.*
*Everywhere we go, anything we touch, you read and you switch*
    *on, it has the message 'STAY ALIVE'.*

*Why we keep quiet rather than speaking.*
*Why don't we go to the clinic to get help. Why don't we go for the*
    *test. Why don't we want to know about our status.*

*THANK U by Mpho M., Gaborone*

The eloquence and feeling of her words profoundly moved me. It was probably the first time I came to realize—and appreciate—the innate wisdom of the people I had naively set out to help. They were not helpless prey: they could be agents of their own salvation. I took her essay to ACHAP, but nothing came of it.

A few months after my first visit, Aaron told me about Pinkie, one of his workers, who had been looking weaker for the last month and had not been at work for over a week. A year earlier, her husband had died from an unknown illness. Aaron suggested that we visit her in Old Naledi, along with his foreman, who knew where Pinkie lived and could help as an interpreter if necessary. A few days later, in the late afternoon, the three of us drove into Old Naledi. Aaron's washed and polished BMW stood out against the brown drabness of the place. The few residents sitting outside in their dirt yards looked with blank indifference at the three of us slowly driving by, the car weaving to avoid particularly large potholes.

The small, one-room house was at the end of a narrow dirt alley, hemmed in by other tiny dwellings. Pinkie was sitting at her doorway. She appeared only mildly malnourished, without the spectral wasting typical of AIDS. In front of her, on a small reed mat in the middle of the alley, lay Comfort, her ten-year-old daughter. Pinkie seemed distracted, and barely evinced a nervous, perfunctory smile when she saw us approaching. Comfort was lying on her side, and was wearing a small pink sun-dress with bright floral patterns. The child was profoundly cachexic, almost skeletal. She stared blankly ahead, too weak even to brush off the flies buzzing and alighting around her eyes and nostrils. Her mother was half-heartedly waving them off with a rolled-up newspaper. It was very hot, and a few neighbors were also sitting outside in the shade, not paying much attention to Pinkie, Comfort, and their uninvited visitors. Sights like Comfort were not new to them, and were best ignored.

The foreman began talking to Pinkie, who smiled back self-consciously. Aaron tersely nodded at his worker, and stood back several steps to give us room, as well as to keep an eye on his car. A few minutes of conversation established the real reason for Pinkie's absence from work: she had been looking after her only child, who had been having diarrhea and fevers. Pinkie had taken Comfort to a local traditional healer, but couldn't afford the "muti," the traditional medicine. She had not taken her to any of the government clinics. When I asked if either of them had been tested for HIV, she looked away and shook her head, embarrassed even to hear the name of the mysterious illness running rampant in her neighborhood.

I gingerly carried Comfort into her house. She felt barely heavier than one of the 30-pound weights I used in the gym. She didn't seem to notice she was being moved. Most of the tiny room was dark and taken up by a king-sized bed, covered with several heavy blankets and pillows. Off to a corner were a small paraffin stove and a very small table, piled with dirty dishes and utensils, flies scavenging the scraps. Two tattered throw rugs were on the dirt floor. There was no sink or bathroom. It was my first exposure to such privation—over the ensuing years I would see similar accommodation over and over again. The room felt like an oven, and the only light came through a small cracked window facing the alley. The foreman accompanied me inside. Pinkie slowly roused herself to follow us into the house.

Gently placing Comfort on the bed, I examined her carefully, as if she were a delicate antique doll. Her stick-like arms and legs had no muscle or fat. Her tongue was coated with thrush, the white fungal infection that is a common marker of advanced HIV disease. My gentle probing had finally animated her, and she began to whimper and reach out for her mother, who was now sitting at the foot of the bed. Pinkie seemed dumbfounded, as if she did not want to know what this was all about. After a minute or so, she reached over and tentatively caressed Comfort's head, but said nothing to her.

Although the foreman assisted with translation, Pinkie understood enough English to answer my questions. Comfort could take liquids, but not solids, probably because of the thrush and being too weak even to chew. The diarrhea had been episodic, usually whenever she would drink liquids. I was already accustomed to the polite, but distant, reserve many Batswana would display with strangers, but I sensed detachment and ambivalence in Pinkie's manner.

I explained that Comfort needed both medicine for her diarrhea and high-calorie liquids for nutrition and hydration. I said I would return in an hour or so with medicines and juices. Given the limitations of Marina Hospital, home care was probably as good as hospitalization, at least for now. I also said that Comfort needed prompt HIV testing, which I would arrange for first thing in the morning. Pinkie took the news passively.

As we left Old Naledi, Aaron was nonplussed by my unease about Pinkie's detachment, her seeming lack of interest in our efforts to help her and her daughter. "She knows if Comfort tests positive, then she has it, too. And she knows her family and neighbors will also know."

An hour later, I drove back alone to their house. Comfort was back outside on the mat, curled up on her side, the flies buzzing about as before. I brought medication for the diarrhea and several large bottles of juice. Pinkie seemed friendlier, and listened closely to my instructions about how Comfort should take the antibiotic and pills for diarrhea.

"She needs to drink as much as possible," I urged. The neighbors watched passively from their front verandas.

"I'll be back tomorrow morning to see how she's doing. We'll take her then for an HIV test." Pinkie showed no reaction to this plan.

The next day, I brought baby food and more juice to Old Naledi. Comfort seemed no worse, and perhaps a bit more alert than the day before. The three of us drove to the Harvard lab at Marina Hospital. Comfort did not even wince at the blood drawing. Holding her in her arms, Pinkie was silent and passive during the trip. Certain that Comfort had AIDS, I also ordered the full array of baseline lab tests necessary before ARVs could be started.

Two days later, the lab results showed no surprises: Comfort was HIV-positive, and her T-cell count abysmally low at ten. That afternoon, I told Pinkie the results. She showed no reaction—no surprise or worry—to the news that Comfort needed to be started on ARVs as soon as possible. Later that afternoon, I pulled some more strings and got her an appointment the next day at the Baylor Children's Clinical Center of Excellence, which provided pediatric AIDS care only to select patients.

Early the next morning, I drove Pinkie and Comfort to the Baylor Clinic. Joining us was Pinkie's older sister, Tsidi, who looked much younger and more prosperous. Friendly and engaging, Tsidi asked questions about her niece's condition and said she had been trying to persuade her sister to get Comfort evaluated. Pinkie, sullen and pouting, sat quietly in the back, while Comfort and her auntie sat in front. On the drive, Tsidi held and caressed her niece, who likewise seemed happy to be with her auntie. It was the first time I saw Comfort smile.

Dedicated earlier in the year, the new Baylor Clinic was as gleaming and spacious as any medical facility in the States. The patient waiting area had tons of toys, and the consultation rooms were clean and well furnished, including computer terminals for retrieving lab tests and recording appointments. Yet despite the large number of infants and children needing AIDS care in Botswana, the Baylor Clinic saw only a fraction of the patients seen in the nearby pediatric AIDS clinic at Marina Hospital. But the facility itself was impressive: foreign visitors hosted by the government were always taken to Baylor, as evidence of Botswana's forward-looking AIDS Programme. I went back to the consultation rooms to thank my pediatric colleague for squeezing Comfort into his schedule.

As I left, I stopped briefly to say goodbye to Comfort, who was still in Tsidi's lap, playing with a plastic duck. Pinkie was reserved, and smiled a weak goodbye. The three of them would take a kombi back to Old Naledi later in the afternoon. It was 8 a.m., and the clinic nurses were calling everyone in the waiting area to group prayer, which probably would be followed by a few hymns, before the clinic session began.

I felt optimistic. In just a few days I'd pulled strings to help one of Aaron's workers. Comfort's pediatrician was kind and competent. An unexpected bonus was Tsidi, who seemed very interested in her niece's well-being. Once Pinkie saw her daughter improve over the coming weeks and months, I thought to myself, she, too, would become more enthusiastic, and might even get HIV tested. Yes, *I was going to save that little girl.* It would require time and patience—it was a simple matter of step A, followed by step B, and so on—but the ARVs were going to work. Comfort would be saved—*her salvation would be a triumph of my will*—and she would become a poster child for the wondrous power of the HIV medicines.

Later that afternoon, I called the pediatrician to see how things went. Because baseline lab tests had already been done, Comfort was started on ARVs that day. Both mother and aunt had been given intensive adherence education, since it was necessary to use liquid preparations of the drugs, which required carefully measuring out exact amounts of each ARV. These dosages would have to be recalculated as Comfort gained weight, until she eventually grew into the standard doses given to adolescents and adults. As part of the visit's routine, the nurses had encouraged Pinkie to be HIV tested, but she adamantly refused, even when Tsidi volunteered to be tested with her. "The mother has some issues," my pediatrician friend concluded. "If we leaned on her any harder, I think she would have refused treatment for Comfort."

"Pinkie's the problem," Aaron mused sadly when he called that evening for an update on the day's events. "She wanted Comfort to die, but then we stepped in. We should have known what we were getting into before we got involved. I wanted to help Pinkie, and instead we got the daughter." I lamely tried to dispute such a bleak assessment, but Aaron, who had lived in Africa all his life, spoke with authority suffused with world-weary compassion.

'"Comfort's an *embarrassment*, a burden to the family. Girls with AIDS are a drain on family resources. Boys they might try to save, but girls have no value. We assumed the mother had AIDS, and now with Comfort, we've gone and proved it. We've created a real mess." Aaron was right: AIDS in Botswana was a "family affair," and the real problem was Pinkie's fear of knowing she herself was HIV-positive. The last thing Pinkie would ever do was tell her co-workers that her daughter was being treated for AIDS, no matter how much the ARVs might help her.

But I remained undeterred. Over the next two weeks, I visited Old Naledi almost daily, bringing juice, candy, baby food, and fruit, which Pinkie eagerly accepted. I always reviewed with her Comfort's medication regimen, which she always said she was giving as ordered. I wanted to believe her, discounting suspicions that Pinkie was telling me what I wanted to hear. On all my visits, I stressed to Pinkie that she needed to be patient, that it would take time for the ARVs to work.

"Within a few months she'll be out playing like any ten-year-old," I promised, perhaps more to myself than her mother. Tsidi called me several times, and reported that she thought her sister was giving Comfort the food and medications, but that she couldn't be certain. Comfort did seem slightly stronger, and at one visit she was sitting up in bed, playing with a doll I had brought her a few days before.

Comfort's follow-up visit to Baylor came two weeks after initiation of the ARVs. My pediatrician friend was pleased with Comfort's progress: she had gained almost two pounds, and seemed more interactive. The clinic nurses felt that Pinkie understood how to give the medicines. According to protocol, a blood count and chemistry were drawn to detect any adverse side-effects of the ARVs, especially anemia from the AZT.

During the two weeks after Comfort's second visit to Baylor, I stopped by Old Naledi only twice each week, figuring that her care would soon settle into a comfortable routine. I also sensed that my daily visits might have been overkill, even patronizing. On these twice-a-week visits, Comfort seemed more alert, and once even smiled when she saw me approaching with more goodies. Pinkie remained largely inscrutable, dutifully reporting that Comfort was "better" and was taking her ARVs. She always appeared removed, even uninterested, and never seemed happy that Comfort was getting better. Perhaps most disconcerting was how Pinkie would never make eye contact with me.

A month after Comfort had been started on treatment, my visit to Old Naledi finally hit the harsh reality of things: the door to the house was closed, locked. No one was at home. A neighbor across the alleyway distractedly volunteered that they had gone to a local traditional healer with the grandmother, who had arrived from their home village. I was stunned, and sensed that things had changed radically.

"Not a good sign," Aaron said that evening, his voice tinged with resignation. "When the grandmother comes, that means the family's decided the child should die in the home village. They went to the sangoma to cure Pinkie of her 'mysterious' infection, and to be told what they wanted to hear, that the child is hopeless and should die. Starvation is the usual way they do it. They put her in a room and she dies a few days later." I struggled to refute such pessimism.

"But Comfort's been doing *better*," I countered, trying to conceal my irritation with my friend's prediction. "She even waved goodbye to me on my last visit there." Aaron sighed charitably at the ignorance and naiveté of his American friend.

"You don't understand. She's an albatross, a burden. They've decided she has to die and there's nothing you or anyone else can do about it. You Americans have this crazy idea about 'the value of each human life,' but it doesn't work that way here. In America they treat a crack addict's 'preemie' that doesn't have a chance of living and spend millions on it, but a child like Comfort would eat up what few resources the family has." I felt punched in the heart, confused and demoralized.

The next morning, I tried to reach Tsidi, but her phone wasn't in service. Late that afternoon, determined not to give in to despair, I returned to Old Naledi. The house was still empty. "Went to Kasane," the same neighbor reported. Kasane was way up north and was probably their home village. Suddenly, I felt foolish—acutely embarrassed—at being there, a self-appointed, putative do-gooder foiled in my clumsy attempt to intervene—or was it interfere?— in the lives of two people I hadn't known, or cared about, until a little over a month earlier. I finally had to admit to myself that I was much more worried about how the failure of my grand gesture might affect my budding friendship with Aaron than I was about the fate of my ten-year-old patient.

Five days later, Tsidi called to report that Comfort had died over the weekend in her home village. The shame has never left me.

---

The very first day I arrived in Botswana, I met Polite, my house-keeper, who lived in a small building behind my three-bedroom house. ACHAP had provided the house, and Polite came with it. It was on a large plot on a quiet residential street in the heart of the capital, surrounded, like all the other houses, by high walls mounted with electric security sensors and razor-sharp barbed wire. The front porch was shaded by several large trees. Every weekday, Polite washed and ironed my clothes, cleaned the dishes, made my bed, carried out the trash, and kept the house clean and in order. It was a luxury I had never had before. My mother was appalled that she even ironed my underwear. Like most Batswana, Polite was always cheerful and, well, polite.

Polite was among the poorest Batswana in Gaborone, with a monthly salary of seven hundred pula, then about 150 dollars, although I always paid her extra. But any way you looked at it, it was essentially slave labor. Polite's chances of being anything other than a domestic were small: her family had no political connections to land her the security of a government job, and her husband worked at a distant wildlife reserve, visiting only a few days a month. More frequent were visits from family and friends, especially Sunday mornings, when they would meet at the front gate and, Bibles in hand, go off to church for the greater part of the day.

Polite always wore on her blouse a prominent, star-shaped silver pin, denoting her membership in the Zion Christian Church, a large evangelical church which had become widespread across southern Africa. Over five million strong, the ZCC was an amalgam of Christian and local beliefs. ZCC pins adorned the lapels and blouses of many people here, including my AIDS patients in the clinics—the stars, doves, and other symbols denoted different levels of faithfulness. At religious gatherings, many of the men wore tan-colored military-style uniforms, decorated with badges signifying various ranks in the church. Older male members would often don large, oversized shoes, painted white—sometimes they would tie onto their shoes fragments of rubber tires that were painted white. This odd shoe style was to allow God to look down and easily identify His people. ZCC members, Polite included, journeyed every Easter to Mount Moria, in South Africa, for a several-day festival of prayer and song. The borders would always be jammed with fleets of kombis and buses, packed with pilgrims besieging the modest immigration posts. Processions of chartered mega-buses whizzed towards the border, the faithful decked out in their white robes and dancing and singing in the aisles, probably all the way to South Africa and back.

Within a few weeks of meeting Polite, it was apparent she was pregnant, already six months along. I really didn't think much about it, since, so I reasoned, it was her business, not mine. She mentioned that she was getting prenatal care at Marina Hospital, barely a ten-minute walk away. A few days after giving birth, she was back in the saddle, ironing my handkerchiefs and underwear. She had a little boy, Paul. When she came back from the hospital, I perfunctorily made over him. He looked like any other newborn: half-human, half-alien. Every morning from Polite's house there would arise the familiar sound of Paul's crying, with its exultation of new life and its attendant promise.

One beautiful Monday morning two months after Paul's birth, as I was sitting on my porch having a second cup of coffee, Polite hurriedly walked up the sidewalk towards me. She usually waited until I left before coming into the house. Cradling Paul in her left arm, she appeared very troubled, with great urgency and worry etched across her usually cheery face. Paul was whimpering softly, as if he, too, sensed something was terribly amiss.

"Dr. Baxter, I have a bad wound inside me." Polite motioned to the front of her chest, where her white blouse was partially open, flapping in the cool breeze. Her ZCC pin dangled haphazardly to the side. She had never complained to me before. Shifting Paul to her other arm, she opened her blouse, revealing shingles over the greater part of the left side of her chest. The angry-looking rash was extensive, going all the way round to her left shoulder-blade area. It was definitely a bad case, and it hurt just to look at the red, weeping vesicles. There were early signs of possible bacterial infection of the raw, denuded skin, with yellowish pus glistening between the zoster lesions. I had never seen such a bad case before.

"A hot fever came on me two days ago, when you were away. I called you, but your phone was off." I had been in Johannesburg for the weekend and had turned off my phone. I felt chastened: while I was playing around in Joburg, my domestic couldn't reach me for help.

"My sister, she said I must go to hospital, but I told her, 'Dr. Baxter will help me when he comes back.'" Paul started to squirm and whimper.

"The pain hurts very bad all night and rises up when I feed Paul. And he doesn't take to the breast like he used to. I pray to God that I am not killing him. I think there is problem with me and Paul, Dr. Baxter, but God is good." Yes, the old "God-is-good" refrain, uttered with half conviction, half-frightened plea, which I had already heard so many times from patients enduring horrendous suffering and privation. The Bible assures us that God knows when even a sparrow falls, and now one of His sparrows had just fallen before me that brilliantly glorious morning.

"Polite, I will help you. Go back to your house and rest. I'll return with medicine." I rushed to the closest chemist for acyclovir for shingles, plus an antibiotic for the bacterial infection and morphine for the pain. One of the great things about being a doctor in Botswana was that you could walk into any pharmacy, show your Botswana medical license, and buy any drug you wanted, including morphine.

As I drove to the pharmacy, I was considering my housekeeper in a completely different light. Polite's shingles almost certainly signified HIV infection. The decreased immunity from HIV allowed the chicken-pox virus which had infected her as a little girl to become reactivated as the localized, painful rash of shingles. In Botswana—in Africa—shingles meant HIV, and Polite probably knew that fact, as did most Batswana, even the ones in the villages. The Setswana word for it was "fire of the gods." Even when it healed, there would often be a permanent scar, sometimes with severe chronic pain. But Polite with shingles and HIV-positive? How could that be? I had never insinuated myself into my housekeeper's private life—I actually knew very little about her.

My hands-off approach to Polite and her family had perturbed Bob, my best friend in New York. When he visited me a few months after I had arrived in Botswana, he met Polite. "You should take Polite and her family out to Sunday dinner every week at the Gab Sun," he remonstrated me many times on that visit and later over the phone. Bob was critical of my studied distance from my housekeeper and her family. But I felt that taking Polite and her family to the buffet at one of the city's first-class hotels would have made her feel uncomfortable. Bob also said I should take the time to read to Vusi, Polite's six-year-old son, who had just started first grade. As well intentioned as my friend was, he didn't realize that in Africa things were different, or at least I thought they were.

Although AIDS surrounded me daily, I was nonetheless dumbfounded that Polite might have it. When I first saw that she was pregnant, I had briefly thought about asking her if she had been HIV tested, but I did not. Crazy as it might have seemed—my naivety back then was astonishing—I felt that, as housekeeper for an AIDS doctor, Polite had somehow bought into the HIV agenda here, that she had absorbed the need for HIV testing, especially during pregnancy, when ARVs could significantly reduce her chances of transmitting HIV to her baby. Because she was getting prenatal care at Marina Hospital, I assumed that they would have counselled her to get HIV tested. What with all of the news and advertisements on every corner, she undoubtedly had heard many times before the whys, wheres, and hows of HIV testing.

As I drove back to the house with the medicines, I tried to rationalize, to excuse my not asking her whether she had been HIV tested. But I could not absolve myself. My reluctance to insert myself into her life had possibly sentenced her son to HIV, and had probably resulted in the suffering and fear she was enduring that very moment. Recalling her words of twenty minutes earlier devastated me: "I pray to God that I am not killing him." She was scared out of her mind that she had infected him.

Medicines in hand, I entered Polite's small house for the first time.

Constructed of large concrete blocks, it was located in the back-most corner of my lot. Unlike the hovels in Old Naledi, it had a proper roof, not one made of sheet metal held down by large boulders. From the outside, it looked more like a large toolshed than a dwelling. Unlike my front yard, the surrounding ground was grassless, and a sole tree next to the house partially shaded three old lounge chairs right outside the entrance. There were two small rooms, one a bedroom and the other a tiny kitchen, separated by a minuscule bathroom. Polite had electricity, but no running water—she had to carry water from the sink attached to the outside of my house. The only visible luxury was a TV in the kitchen, a hand-me-down from my friend Aaron.

Polite was lying on a bright quilt on the bed, which, except for a small bedside table, took up the entire room. Paul was lying next to her, sleeping, and Vusi, her six-year-old, was quietly sitting next to his baby brother. He looked worried, warily watching his mother and the elderly doctor who lived in the big house next to his.

I went over with Polite how to take her medicine. On second inspection, the shingles looked even worse. I knew it would take weeks to resolve, and even then there'd probably be a large permanent scar. Although it was too early to ask—there was no urgency from a clinical viewpoint—I had to know.

"Polite, did you have the HIV test done when you had Paul?" I immediately realized I should have phrased the question better. "I mean, have you ever had the HIV test?"

Polite seemed embarrassed, ashamed. In Botswana, shame and guilt had darkened everything associated with HIV—being tested, not being tested, living with HIV, dying with HIV. "No," she answered softly, averting her eyes. There was no point in pressing the issue just then—that discussion could wait.

Fear and stigma associated with "the HIV test" were all-pervasive in Botswana. Daily, scores of patients would be admitted to hospitals across the country with life-threatening AIDS-related diseases, but most of them would still adamantly refuse the HIV test. People would sooner go to their graves than agree to the HIV test.

The reasons for this fear and stigma had eluded everyone here, and already a small fortune had been spent on various research studies, mostly by Westerners, to unlock the secret, to find the magic bullet to get people to come forward and be tested. Prior to AIDS, the Batswana had enjoyed a very enlightened and healthy attitude towards sex. Sexually transmitted diseases and pregnancy out of wedlock evoked little, if any, opprobrium. When the West brought in its HIV drugs, fear of espousing a double standard caused us also to import American obsession with confidentiality and "AIDS exceptionalism." The Setswana word for "confidential" implied secrecy, a need to hide something shameful. The West's legalistic penchant for "pre-test" and "post-test" counselling had been taken to ridiculous extremes here: the length and solemnity of such counselling by nurses and social workers in the clinics frightened away many people. After such a scary discussion, only hardy souls would have the courage to get the test, let alone return in two weeks for the result.

The Botswana government itself had also been responsible for the demonization of the HIV test. Several years earlier, with the best of intentions, President Mogae had declared it the "patriotic duty" of young Batswana to remain HIV-negative. The unfortunate implication, of course, was that citizens who became HIV infected had somehow disgraced their country, their village, and their family. The sick joke was that the easiest way for a Motswana to remain HIV-negative was not to get tested. Vice-President Ian Khama made it even worse when he was quoted in the newspapers as saying that people on HIV medications had been, by their "immoral behaviors," draining the country of precious resources. Hellfire-and-brimstone condemnations emanated every Sunday from many pulpits in the country.

Fear of the HIV test had impacted national security as well. The BDF—the Botswana Defense Force—had realized early on that mandatory HIV testing would seriously affect recruitment for this all-volunteer army. Instead, unknown to most applicants, a screening T-cell count—a measure of immune strength—was done as a surrogate HIV test, allowing the BDF to reject those with low counts. This subterfuge had its limitations, since applicants recruited with normal T-cell counts could still be infected and later succumb to the disease. Estimates of the percentage of soldiers who were in fact HIV-positive had always been classified. In his addresses to new recruits, President Mogae would exhort them to practice safe sex, for the sake of the country. Imagine President George W. Bush giving similar advice to West Point cadets.

I always discussed HIV testing at the KITSO course, the country's three-day HIV training for health care workers here. "How dare you," I would exhort the attendees, "tell your patients to get tested when you yourself don't!" Some of the attendees—the nurses more so than the doctors— would appear to understand this finger-to-the-heart admonition, and would smile back nervously. Several months after arriving in Botswana, I befriended a young Motswana woman who worked at my bank. She always helped me with wiring money to the States. Spunky, buxom, and full of life, she once told me the sad story of her mother, who had worked as an HIV counsellor for her local village, urging her countrymen to be tested. She had died a few years earlier from a mysterious illness, never tested for HIV. My friend assured me that she herself tested regularly, but I often wondered.

I told Polite I would check in on her later in the day. As always, she thanked me and started to apologize for not being able to work then. I would hear nothing of it. "Forget about the house and the laundry. I want you to rest!"

By the time I returned home, it was nearly six o'clock. The sun was already low in the sky, and distant thunderclouds, which less than an hour earlier had been formidable and menacing, were rapidly fading into nothingness. I rushed to see Polite, fearing that, as with Comfort a few months earlier, I would find that she, too, had disappeared, taken away to her home village, to die from her own "mysterious illness." But there was Vusi playing with some rope in the yard, and Polite's younger sister, a frequent overnight guest, sitting nearby, peeling potatoes over a bowl in her lap. Polite was awake in her bed, with little Paul asleep beside her. She smiled and tried to sit up when she saw me. She still appeared weak and very uncomfortable from the "wound" on her chest. Yet she carried still another, even greater worry.

"Sir, they won't pay me if I do not work at your house! They said they will send another person." It was an all-too-common worry of the working poor here: if you cannot work, you will be replaced. Many times in the clinics, I had heard similar stories. A patient with AIDS would be sacked as an au pair for a diplomat's household, even though she might be recovering on ARVs. A manual laborer, weakened from TB, would lose his construction job, because high unemployment among unskilled workers guaranteed that there would always be someone to take his place. There was no such thing as "light duty" until medications restored a patient's health. These unlucky people had no choice but to return to their families in their home villages, where access to medical care was often limited. Even workers whose employers allowed them time off to go to the HIV clinics for medical care could ill afford to take off the entire day and wait in long queues to see the doctor, or to collect their medicines from the pharmacy. For most people here, a "sick day" was a "no pay" day. I didn't know whether Polite's fears were justified, whether ACHAP—an AIDS relief program designed for people exactly like her—would continue to pay her while she recovered.

"I must be your housekeeper, or I have nowhere to live," Polite added, with neither fear nor anger. "But God is good." Polite sounded resigned, but remained steadfast in the belief that, circumstances notwithstanding, God would look after her.

"Polite, everything will be OK. The important thing is that we get you feeling better." I again inspected the wide swathe of chest and upper back which the shingles virus had denuded, and then reapplied clean dressing. Gone were Polite's becalming smile and cheerfulness, which had previously seemed innate. The most urgent issue was preventing a secondary bacterial infection from setting in. Another concern was to stave off post-herpetic neuralgia, the chronic, often severe pain that could linger for years after the shingles lesions had healed. I again went over her medicines with her, and said I would look in on her the next day.

"I'm not going to let anything bad happen to you. I promise." Many black Africans had heard similar promises over the past 500 years from white people, often voiced with the same urgency and conviction. Sometimes the promises had even been kept. "And I absolutely forbid you to go to your home village without first checking with me—do you understand?" I was pleading, not commanding.

"Yes, sir," was Polite's only reply, pressured and distracted in tone, and not her typical, effusive "Thank you, sir!"

The next day I called ACHAP. They already knew about Polite's plight—in Botswana it was impossible to keep anything secret—and they gave me the good news. I rushed home after work to tell her.

"ACHAP says it will pay you while you're sick, even if it takes several weeks. And of course, I'll still pay you the usual extra. They said they'd send someone to take your place while you're off." Polite seemed relieved but also a little annoyed at hearing someone else would be caring for her doctor. As housekeeper, she regarded my residence as "her house," for which she was responsible. She did not like the idea of a total stranger taking her place. Just then, I spied Polite's mother in the adjacent kitchen, laboring over a pot of porridge on the small stove. A quiet, elderly lady, the mother had visited from time to time, but today her appearance alarmed me.

"Polite, you're not going to go to your home village, are you? We can get you better," I pleaded, "but only if you stay here."

"You are my doctor who helps me with my wound," she answered confidently. "I tell my mother, 'Dr. Baxter will look after Paul and me. He says I will be better here.' God is good to give me you."

The next morning, I briefly looked in on Polite. The pain was less, and the first signs of healing had appeared, although it would take weeks for recovery. Polite was more concerned about who ACHAP would be sending that day to work in her place. The usual custom would have been for Polite to recruit someone she knew, preferably a family member, to fill in for her. But her supervisor at ACHAP had other plans and, most likely, relatives of her own who needed work. She told me that a woman named Doreen would be coming.

Arriving home that evening, I found my new temporary house-keeper still at work—Polite always finished her chores well before I returned. Doreen was engrossed in ironing a shirt on the ironing board set up in the living room. There was an earnest desperation about her as she labored to remove creases she had imprinted into them, probably for the twentieth time. Forlornly hanging from a nearby curtain rod was another hopelessly creased shirt, which may or may not have been ironed. They reminded me of my ill-fated efforts many decades earlier in medical school to iron my shirts myself. A very young woman, Doreen appeared flustered when she saw me.

"Dr. Baxter?"

I smiled and nodded affirmation.

"Dr. Baxter, I've never been a maid before!" Her voice had a plaintive, desperate tone. "I'm sorry, but I can't iron." It appeared that Doreen had been wrestling with the ironing for most of the afternoon.

"I thought ACHAP said you'd worked as a housekeeper before."

"*Oh no*, Dr. Baxter," she answered with half-amazement. "I worked as a cleaner at the airport. I've never been a maid before." I stared dumbly at her, more out of pity than annoyance.

"Doreen, don't worry about it. We'll manage. Look, all I need is for you to wash the dishes and my clothes. You don't need to make the bed or clean anywhere, just change the bed once a week. As for ironing, you'll just have to keep at it. You'll learn." Doreen appeared unconvinced about this, and from her efforts thus far, I was, too. "Now just go home. It's late. Finish the ironing tomorrow."

"But Dr. Baxter, Polite will cane me if she sees creased shirts! She told me so today! That one, she looked very mad at me." Doreen, who was much younger than Polite, seemed genuinely concerned.

"Go, now!" I benignly commanded her. Happy to be sent home without being sacked—or caned—Doreen said nothing, and within seconds was on her way out. I retreated to Polite's house, to see how she was doing. Not very well as it turned out, and not because of her shingles.

"Dr. Baxter, *that girl* can't iron!" Polite was seething in her disdain. The tone of "that girl" was the same used by clinic nurses annoyed and frustrated with recalcitrant patients. "She has been ironing for all afternoon and they all have creases!" Doreen was probably lucky to have got off the property alive.

"Don't worry," I replied, "you'll be back to ironing soon, but you need to rest for now. If I have to, I can do the ironing myself." Polite looked mightily confused at the thought of her doctor doing his own ironing.

Over the next two weeks, Polite slowly improved, growing stronger and experiencing much less pain. Amazingly, Doreen also improved in her ironing, thanks to Polite's mentoring—once they started talking to one another, they found that they were related, sharing nearby home villages. Soon they were sharing lunch together. A month after Polite fell sick, Doreen returned to her job at the airport, armed with the new and saleable skill of shirt ironing.

The following week, I told Polite I was taking her and her boys to Marina to be tested for HIV. There were no protests, no procrastinations. As we were going back to the house, I told her that

I was pretty sure she was positive. The big question was whether Paul was spared or not. Her older boy was probably OK, since he hadn't been sick and looked perfectly normal, although sometimes infected kids—Comfort was probably an example—can go on for many years before succumbing to the virus.

A week later the results came back: Polite and her baby were both positive, the older boy negative. My not asking her six months earlier about her HIV status when she was pregnant had allowed a little baby to become HIV infected. When I told her the test results, she cried as she held both of her sons to her bosom.

I held her hand and assured her that everything would be all right, that I would help her. And I did. Her T-cell count was in the mid-three hundreds, well above the two hundred count where she would be eligible for treatment in government clinics. But I pulled strings and got her and Paul on treatment a week later.

Over the ensuing six years, Polite and her family flourished. Polite didn't have the guilt and shame so many others had about their infection—she told others to be HIV tested, and even was featured in an article in ACHAP's newsletter. After a while I stopped berating myself whenever she proclaimed how I had saved her and Paul, how God had sent me to them. I had reached the point in my life where I was resolved to learn from my screw-ups and not wallow in guilt.

Doctors make lots of mistakes, but Polite was one of my biggest: an AIDS doctor who couldn't bring himself to ask his pregnant maid to get HIV tested, all because he didn't want to intrude, because he was too polite.

———

The catastrophes of Comfort and Polite starkly drove home how I could no longer hide in my bedroom, hermetically sealed off, taking refuge in the so-called life-affirming lessons I had brought with me from the States. When I came to Botswana with all of my good intentions, I thought I had all the answers, but my hubris had probably cost a little girl her life and my aloofness had allowed a baby to become HIV infected. I thought I had all the answers, but Comfort and Polite showed that I didn't even know the right questions to ask, let alone the answers.

I had to start over from scratch.

Somehow sensing that Botswana's time and space would save me, I persevered and plunged into a whirlpool of activities: teaching HIV medicine to the healthcare workers, volunteering at the local hospice, going on "outreach" visits to surrounding villages, and eventually becoming a respected expert to whom people turned for advice. I had so much to learn over the subsequent six years.

# Chapter 6

## Learning to Dance

I never could dance—it just wasn't in my genes. The Church of Christ in my small hometown in rural Ohio regarded dancing as on par with smoking and drinking, something that risked impure thoughts or worse. True, at 4-H camp I did join in the evening square-dancing, but dosidoing wasn't like twisting and gyrating your body, Elvis- or Beetles-style, at the high school prom. When I was a young doctor in West Virginia, a friend—a flamboyant hairdresser of note—tried to teach me, but I was hilariously hopeless. I just couldn't relax and not worry about what people thought. But if I have ever come close to letting go, to dancing and shaking my aged bones in front of other people, it was in Botswana, whenever I was standing before thirty to forty healthcare workers in the KITSO course, teaching, joking, bantering, and just letting them know that, yes, they could do it, they could treat HIV patients.

Right after the debacles of Comfort and Polite, I sought sanctuary, if you will, as "lead trainer" of KITSO, the country's three-day course on the nuts and bolts of HIV care. Initially, I was just one of several instructors, but, busy as the others were with their research or administrative duties, they were happy to cede the main role to me. I regained my stride in KITSO, which I would lead almost weekly, ultimately training several thousand healthcare workers—social workers, lab technicians, pharmacists, nurses, and doctors. Before a clinic could start treating patients, the staff had to pass the KITSO course. The healthcare workers didn't mind having to take the course: government employees, in fact, loved the various catered workshops and in-service meetings that let them escape the tedium of their jobs.

"Kitso" is Setswana for "knowledge," the acronym contorted into "Knowledge, Innovation, and Training Shall Overcome AIDS." Its multi-layered structure, like everything else in the Treatment Programme, made it difficult to determine who was actually in charge. The government contracted with Harvard to develop and present it, ACHAP funded it, and the Ministry of Health reviewed its results. The Botswana-Harvard Partnership was always the elephant in the room, a behemoth which everyone needed—its large modern lab building at Marina Hospital was truly imposing—but which everyone loved to criticize, simply because it was so big. Its lab and research studies trained and employed hundreds of Batswana, and if it weren't for its doctors and Batswana nurses, the Treatment Programme would have been delayed for many months, at the cost of many lives. Everyone loved Harvard's competence and payroll but railed about its presumed power, and there were periodic spats between Harvard and ACHAP. The politics could often turn ugly: there were several times when we didn't know if there would be money for the next week's KITSO course. After heads were knocked together, ACHAP would come through with the money. I don't think Bill Gates would have approved of all the petty bickering. But he definitely got his money's worth from KITSO.

Held in a variety of venues, almost all of them cramped and dingy, the three-day course consisted of eleven lectures and was as non-technical as possible, since, as I would always tell my students, HIV treatment wasn't brain surgery.

"It's not that I'm smarter than you, it's just that I'm older," I would encourage them. I would tell them about the turf battles we had had in the States several years earlier over whether only infectious disease specialists could treat HIV, and how we soon learned that practically anyone could do it.

At first, the KITSO courses were held in Gaborone, but after the first year, as ARV rollout progressed, we took the show on the road, first to the towns and then the outermost villages. When I taught in Gumare, an isolated post up north, I had to take care driving to and from the course, since elephants, including massive, aggressive bulls, would blithely saunter across the road. That was the same time my car got stuck in the sand on my first night there as I was driving to the remote game lodge where I was staying. I was totally stranded—there was no cellphone service. If it wasn't for my friend Aaron calling the lodge to see if I had arrived safely, I would have had to spend the cold night in my car, surrounded by wild animals.

But regardless of where it was held, every KITSO course started with a prayer. Not asking for an opening prayer or hymn would have been a major faux pas. I preferred a hymn, which always had a haunting, otherworldliness to it—the students all seemed to know whatever hymn someone started to belt out. And how they could sing! The Batswana were, so it seemed, born with melodic voices, further refined by years of singing in church. Most of the attendees, especially the women, dressed in their Sunday finest.

After the opening prayer or hymn, I would always write my mobile phone number on the flip chart in front of the class. "You can reach me any time of the day or night you have any clinical questions, be they HIV-related or non-HIV-related. I'd love to hear from you!" And call me they did, often with stories of unfathomable woe, but usually ending with "but God is good."

I invented colorful analogies and metaphors to clarify abstract topics, and they understood most of them, since they were immersed in Western pop culture. So they immediately got it when, in the lecture on immunity, I referred to the T-cell as "The Terminator cell, the Arnold Schwarzenegger cell, which blasts away at infections." I felt as if I was a nightclub performer, refining and perfecting my act, thinking up new routines to keep things fresh and stop me from getting in a rut. As they laughed at my jokes, they learned a lot of HIV medicine.

KITSO gave me special insights into Botswana and its people. There was their adamant refusal to accept the African origins of HIV. I tried mightily to get them to realize that their near-apoplectic reaction to this fact illustrated the shame and guilt invested in HIV, but they wouldn't listen. They were absolutely shocked when I proclaimed that sexual kissing was safe. Many attendees, mostly the men, insisted that HIV-infected women should be barred from having babies—oh, how the women, glowering their disapproval, would arch their backs at the men on this issue. Pointing out how gender inequality had fueled the spread of HIV, I challenged the men on this matter, to the approving nods of the women. They resolutely insisted that homosexuality was a Western disorder not present in Botswana—after a while, I didn't even go there anymore. I would exhort them to give targeted safe-sex messages to patients— a condom for rectal and vaginal sex, every time, no exceptions—and to avoid a "total-body-condom" approach, which would only cause people to ignore safe-sex messages, especially the younger ones who always felt they'd live forever anyway.

Early on, Dr. Ndwapi told me one of the little-appreciated problems with prevention messages in Botswana. The phrase "condoms all of the time," when translated into Setswana, could also be interpreted as "condoms *some* of the time." "It's a relative thing," Ndwapi explained. "'Always' in Setswana just means more often than 'none of the time,' so it can come across as meaning 'use condoms more often than none of the time,' which can mean just 'some of the time.'" I wondered if the CDC and UNAIDS knew this fact in their ongoing search for the magic bullet, the right words to get the Batswana to use condoms.

A recurring question my students always had was whether the Treatment Programme was sustainable, whether they were being led along by the West, only to be abandoned someday. This, of course, was an understandable concern, given what the colonial powers had done in the past to Africa and what the new quasi-colonial powers—the drug companies and Western aid organizations—might do in the future. I reminded them that well over 80 per cent of the cost of the Treatment Programme was borne by the government, and that Botswana had already developed enough expertise to carry on with the Programme alone. "We've crossed a line here, and we can't go back. Bottom line: you're not going to be abandoned." History has proven me right.

I didn't have to convince them that the ARVs worked, that the Treatment Programme wasn't a scam concocted by the drug companies to bamboozle Africans. That sort of rubbish had been government policy in neighboring South Africa. I loved to praise the political leadership of Botswana—President Mogae in particular—for having the courage to launch the Treatment Programme. "If the Minister of Health here in Botswana spouted the sort of nonsense being bandied about in South Africa, the President would hand the Minister his head on a silver platter," I would half joke, since he probably would. Most of my students had already seen friends and neighbors—indeed, themselves—recover on ARVs.

I repeatedly challenged them to re-examine the psychosocial implications of HIV infection, particularly stigma. Safer-sex messages in Botswana, as in the West, had been hijacked by the moralists, people who labelled HIV a "behavioral disease." I always bristled at this phrase, since it perpetuated stigma. "I don't like to look on HIV as a 'behavioral disease,'" I would tell my students.

"Do we think of lung cancer, diabetes, or heart disease as primarily 'behavioral diseases?' Do we demonize smokers and obese people for having lung cancer, heart disease, and diabetes the way we look down on people with HIV for having unsafe sex? All this talk about 'good' behavior and 'bad' behavior risks moral judgements and censure, and leads to people being categorized as 'good' and 'bad' according to their sexual activities. This is how stigma happens, and it's stigma that's keeping people from coming forward to be tested and causing them to die in their home villages of a 'mysterious illness.'" At the very least, I may have mitigated the shame many of my HIV-infected students felt, and perhaps even made the others look on HIV in an entirely new light.

To keep my students awake—many of the venues had no air conditioning during the hot summers—I shared the ironies of medicine from my own career. "I remember when I was a medical student on a dermatology rotation in the early 1970s. One day the derm resident came to us all excited. 'Guys, there's a patient here who has something you'll never see again.' So we followed him into one of the rooms, and there was an old man sitting in a chair, and the resident pointed out a dark-purple spot on his foot. 'This is Kaposi's sarcoma,' the resident told us with great satisfaction. *'You'll never see another case like this for the rest of your career!'*" The attendees smiled at the irony, since AIDS-related KS was rampant in Botswana.

One of the lectures everyone was keen to hear was the prevention of mother-to-child transmission of HIV, or PMTCT. Stopping such transmission had been one of the major goals of the Treatment Programme, but many expectant mothers still refused to be HIV tested, despite intensive counselling. Whenever I gave this lecture, my mind would wander back to Polite, who most likely had been counseled repeatedly on her prenatal visits at Marina. Why she had refused would probably never be fully known, even to her. "It was with PMTCT we had the first ray of hope in this epidemic," I would always start this lecture. "I remember, it was in 1995 when the AIDS

Clinical Trial 076 first showed that AZT could reduce mother-to-child transmission from 25 percent to 8 percent, and we all rejoiced that we could actually stop this virus from infecting babies."

Part of the PMTCT lecture dealt with infant feeding options, a subject of intense debate and research in Africa. Ideally, to prevent HIV transmission through breast milk, all HIV-positive mothers should formula-feed their babies, but in Africa things were not always so simple. For one thing, there was stigma: formula-feeding your baby was announcing to everyone in your family and village that you were HIV-positive. Many mothers did not disclose their infection to their partners, out of fear of abandonment, beatings, or worse. Then there was the problem of obtaining clean water for mixing the formula, as well as perennial problems with the adequate supply of formula, too often due to government incompetence. Only many years later would we learn that ARVs for the mother would prevent HIV transmission from breast milk.

Perhaps nothing gave me greater appreciation of the special genius of the Batswana than the session on case studies on the final afternoon of the course. They would break up into small groups to discuss real-life patient cases assigned to them. In the tradition of the *kgotla*—the gathering of the entire village, under the leadership of the local chief—the participants eagerly engaged one another in animated discussion of their group's case. The Batswana loved to discuss and debate, and it was unusual for a group not to get caught up in its particular case. At the end of the group session, the group leaders—they were usually evenly divided between doctors and nurses—presented the cases, summarizing each group's approach to its particular patient case. There was one which I will always remember. The case itself was pretty simple and was intended to test their knowledge of the common side effects of one of the ARVs, efavirenz (EFV):

"A twenty-five-year-old man was started two weeks ago on AZT/3TC/EFV, with baseline CD4 count of thirty and viral load of 250,000. He comes in now complaining about dizziness, vivid dreams, and one episode of 'strange behavior.' He is very frightened, and says he is taking his medicine exactly as prescribed."

I was mesmerized by the confident authority of the young woman, a nurse, who came forward to present her group's management of this case. Silly me, I had expected only a few sentences about the well-known side effects of EFV.

"This twenty-five-year-old-man was in the prime of his life. He went to Tebelopele [the national HIV testing site] to prove to himself that he was negative. He had told his girlfriend that he had never practiced unsafe sex, but he knew that several years ago, when he was wild and into drugs, he had had unsafe sex. When he got the results, he was devastated. He thought he would lose his good job as a restaurant manager and that his girlfriend, who came from a prominent family, would leave him. He went to a traditional healer, but he started to get sicker with fevers and night sweats. He went to church and prayed for a miracle, but he did not know that the miracle was already here with the ARVs. He finally confided in his grandmother, who told him to go to the ARV clinic at Marina. Grandma went with him as his adherence partner. The side effects went away, and several months later he was feeling much better. He told his family and girlfriend, who accepted him. His job was not affected, and when he finally told his co-workers, some of them came forward to be tested and to get into treatment."

I was dumbstruck, blown away by the way she had constructed a real-life case out of the question, ending on a note of hope. Perhaps there was more truth to her story than she let on.

While teaching KITSO, I forgot my cares and no longer felt a lonely outsider in Africa. Every group was different, but I felt a special connection with all of them. After every course ended, I would feel sad, as each group *had given so much to me*, and I would always remark to my friends how absolutely wonderful my latest batch of students was. Over 95 percent of the attendees passed the KITSO test, held the day after the last lecture, granting them the much-coveted KITSO certificate. At the end of the test, they were asked to complete a course evaluation. One of them wrote: "Dr. Baxter has given unto me a lamp, which will allow me to light the way for people living with AIDS." Another asked if I was married, and a third enquired if I did wedding parties.

Ten years later, on my second sojourn in Botswana, people would still approach me in restaurants, in grocery stores, almost anywhere, and proudly introduce themselves as having been one of my KITSO students. I would always ask what they were now doing, and add apologetically, "I can't remember your name, but I do remember your smile." And I would always thank them for saying hello. The Batswana valued the certificates they got from their various workshops and conferences, and I am certain that even today, in someone's office or home, there is a framed KITSO certificate on the wall, signed by me.

And I never again felt self-conscious about dancing, or at least trying.

# Chapter 7

# Outreach 2003:
# Molepolole

One of the pleasing things about language is how certain words are fun to say over and over, playfully rolling off your tongue. For me, Molepolole—Mo'-lay-po-lo'-lay—is one of them, sounding much like the incantations of the witch doctors practicing their trade there. In addition to having the largest number of such traditional healers, Molepolole reportedly had the highest number of lightning strikes—witch doctors were believed to use lightning as retribution, especially in retaliation for curses such as AIDS, which other witch doctors had put on people. Although its name might sound exotic—like Casablanca, Marrakesh, or Katmandu—Molepolole was anything but, as I would soon learn on my first "outreach" visit to its hospital, soon after the debacles of Comfort and Polite.

Molepolole was the first time I ventured outside of the capital. For nearly six months, I had been holed up in Gaborone, a city of 600,000—not counting illegal Zimbabweans—which really didn't feel like a city, let alone a residence for over half a million souls. In fact, Gaborone really didn't feel like much of anything, so spread out and, well, boring it was. But better quiet and boring than dangerous and crowded like other African capitals.

Molepolole was Botswana's largest village, with a population of around 64,000, not counting goats, cows, chickens, wild donkeys, and stray dogs. On my maiden drive there, only an hour from Gaborone, I took in the immensity of the countryside for the first time: bleak, brown, solitary, unredeemed by the glare of the early morning sunshine. The landscape was flat and monotonous, with squat trees and drab, low-lying bush. Monumental termite hills—each an insect universe unto itself—erupted off the roadside, often taller than the trees. The uniform scenery was occasionally punctuated with lonely cattle posts, isolated one-room huts, and forlorn roadside stops, where a few people waiting for a bus would valiantly try to flag down a ride. The two-lane asphalt road was maintained well enough to render it very dangerous—drivers here were notoriously reckless. Although the road was largely empty, I carefully kept to the speed limit. A few weeks earlier, I had gotten my first speeding ticket in Gaborone. Like a fool, I paid the 100 pula fine to the policeman, instead of at the Central Police Station, which is what the cop should have told me to do. Five years earlier, Sweden, earnestly intent as only the Swedes can be, donated speed radar guns, which the police actually used, especially towards the end of their pay periods. However, the Swedes crossed the line a few years later when they threw in free alcohol breathalyzers: one of the first drunks pulled over was an important government minister. After that, the breathalyzers were quickly put in permanent storage.

But obeying the speed limit was no guarantee you'd survive the roads, even if there wasn't a driver in sight. There were always fearsome potholes lurking around the bend, threatening to tear your tires and wheels apart, or worse. Goats, cattle, and wild donkeys grazed placidly at the roadside, but when you least expected it, they'd decide to blithely meander to the other side. Hitting a cow at full speed was a ticket to the afterlife. Already I'd learned the driving maxim about animals here: "Heads down, OK to go; heads up, go slow." Today the assorted livestock seemed content to munch on what little grass there was, heads down.

As I tooled along in my white Toyota Corolla—a model as ubiquitous here as wild donkeys—the emptiness of the countryside opened to the blue horizon, and the blazing overhead sun left no shadow for escape from the immense, engulfing void. And if you weren't at peace with yourself, "There was no joy in the brilliance of sunshine," as Conrad's Marlow had said.

Closer to the village outskirts, the road deteriorated into gargantuan potholes, their jagged, crumbling edges sometimes forcing me to swerve into the other lane. As I drove deeper into the village, the previous solitude gradually morphed into the frantic, frenetic life of an African town. The roadside now teemed with people walking to and fro, some balancing bags and boxes on their heads—one elderly woman carried on hers a car's entire exhaust system, nearly twice as long as she was tall. Swarms of kombis and taxis erratically swerved on and off the road to pick up and disgorge passengers. As the narrow road snaked into the heart of the village, traffic ground down to bumper-to-bumper, lurching forward at slow speeds. "Downtown" Molepolole was a dense hodgepodge of small grocery stores, butcheries, hardware stores, discount furniture suppliers, take-away eateries, a Barclays Bank, churches, tire repair shops, a few private medical clinics, several offices of traditional healers, and the police station. All the while, herds of goats and cattle carried on with wayward abandon, in perfect concert with the helter-skelter chaos of pedestrians, taxis, and kombis. The sun blazing overhead seemed to boil the village's activities to fever pitch. The dust kicked up by all the human and animal activity created a scrim of glowing autumnal colors.

Like everywhere else, I didn't feel conspicuous or out of place, least of all in any danger, other than of running over someone's goat or elderly grandmother. Older Batswana largely regarded whites with a combination of tolerance, bemusement, and pity. "Vomit from the sea"—that was the literal Setswana translation for us white people, the strange beings washed in with the ocean's foam centuries ago.

After what seemed like an eternity, I finally reached Scottish Livingstone Hospital, on the other side of town. Set back from the main road, the hospital was approached by a long, winding driveway, unpaved and rutted with deep potholes. The hospital looked as if it hadn't been renovated since its founding by missionaries from Scotland a century ago. As with many African hospitals, it was a spread-out array of a dozen or so one-story wards and office blocks, all interconnected by walkways with overhead canopies of rusted corrugated metal. Dozens of cars and pick-up trucks were parked haphazardly around some of the buildings, many with patients stretched out in the back beds, waiting for their appointments.

Parking far enough away so I wouldn't be blocked in later, I headed for the clinic. A multitude of patients and their families were sitting on the grounds and under the covered passageways, competing for precious shade from the sun. The sicker patients lay on mats and blankets, with nearby relatives waving off flies. A few of the weakest ones were on hospital gurneys, curled up in the fetal position, their skeletal frames disappearing into the folds of their blankets. Although it was already warm outside, the majority of people were still in overcoats and hats, since dawn was chilly this time of year. Most of the patients had arrived here many hours ago, well before sunrise.

The AIDS clinic was a new, prefabricated building which housed five consultation rooms, a pharmacy, a tiny nursing station, and a small waiting area. Patients and family members, some standing, others sitting, blocked the entrance, and spilled onto the narrow sidewalk outside. I slowly pushed my way through the throng blocking the doorway, much like getting onto a crowded New York City subway, except that here they politely gave way to the old white man. Just inside the door, off to the side, a nurse was methodically weighing patients as they entered, marking the result on their patient cards. In the waiting area, people occupied every square inch of every bench, including those lining the narrow hallway leading to the exam rooms. The weaker ones were lying on the floor, further adding to the congestion. Some people were merely waiting for refills of their ARVs—even though patients already on treatment might see the doctor only every three months, they still had to return monthly for refills, often from distant villages. Other patients were waiting to see the nurses for group counselling on ARV adherence prior to their appointments. And still others were there only to see the doctor. Some of the people crowded into the waiting area were family members or friends—the Treatment Programme strongly encouraged patients to bring along "adherence partners," to assist them in taking their ARVs. The room had the familiar, musky odor of humanity in close quarters—not of unwashed bodies, but of human beings thrown together in the struggle for survival. On the wall in a distant corner was a small box marked "Suggestions."

As with all the other AIDS clinics across Botswana, the patients were not waiting in silence. This was not the typical waiting area of an AIDS clinic in America, where patients, averting their eyes from fellow sufferers, sat in studied silence, and the staff spoke in hushed tones. Rather, the waiting area of the Molepolole AIDS clinic was an open forum for free exchange of information among the assembled. Amid the cacophony of voices were personal testimonials to the efficacy of the ARVs, advice about medication side effects, news of the arrival of a new traditional healer from Malawi, opinions about which doctors and nurses were nice and which were not, and details of upcoming church revival meetings. Everything was being bantered back and forth among friends, neighbors, and total strangers. Such transparency—this sense of shared community—was typical of the Batswana, whose traditions had centered for innumerable generations on the kgotla, where everyone discussed issues of common import.

I stopped at the nursing station to greet the nurses and introduce myself. Coming to a hospital or clinic for the first time without introducing yourself was a major lapse of protocol—the Batswana were always polite, but took offence if you appeared to slight them, no matter how good your intentions might be. The real powers in the clinics and hospitals were the matrons and nurses, addressed as "sister." Flattering them was always a good idea.

"Sisters, you all look so young, and I feel so old!"

"Oh, Dr. Baxter," one of them half-flirted, "in Botswana, a man becomes old only when he dies!"

"Now I know why I like Botswana so much!" Smiles all round. One of the nurses directed me to the doctor's office.

I navigated my way down the narrow hallway to the consultation rooms. Both sides of the passageway were lined with narrow wooden benches, on which patients perched, carefully monitoring their place in the queue. Today I was sitting in with Dr. Moyo, one of my first KITSO students, who was from Zimbabwe, and who had been working at Scottish for almost two years. Many of the doctors in Botswana were not Batswana, and had to be recruited from other African countries.

This morning, Dr. Moyo had already started seeing patients. I sat off to the side, out of the way. On initial inspection, the consultation room appeared much like any medical examination room in the West, with the requisite desk, chairs, examination table, and washbasin. However, there was no medical equipment anywhere, and the exam table was covered with one folded sheet, which would serve all the several dozen patients seen that day. Taped on the wall next to the doctor's desk was a hand-drawn graph, showing how the inexorable decline in the T-cell count was associated with various opportunistic infections. Such visual aids helped patients better understand the risk of AIDS and the hope offered by ARVs.

On the other walls were large glossy posters, produced by the Ministry of Health, showing cheerful, healthy Batswana exhorting their countrymen about safer sex, HIV testing, and ARV medication adherence. One poster featured a simple visual representation of how HIV targets T-cells: the T-cell count was represented as cattle within the fences of a cattle post, with ferocious lions—HIV—waiting outside. Some well-meaning Westerners branded such simplistic illustrations as patronizing, but time to explain abstract concepts was always in short supply at the clinics, as hordes of patients were clamoring for a life raft.

As I settled into my chair, Dr. Moyo's nurse was in the middle of explaining to a patient how to take the ARVs. Nurses were crucial to HIV care here, often serving as translators, since many of the doctors didn't know Setswana, a very descriptive, metaphorical language, imbued with powerful cultural nuances, which an outsider like me could never fully understand. I was always fascinated how a simple question, such as "Have you had any fevers or sweats?" would elicit an animated five-minute discussion in Setswana between patient and nurse, eventually concluding with a simple "yes" or "no" reply from the nurse. Even more important than being translators, nurses were teachers and mentors for their patients, who, after all, were often friends, neighbors, and even relatives. The nurses were helpful in assessing whether or not a patient was ready to start ARV treatment, and I almost always followed their advice in this regard. The nurses were also responsible for adherence education, which was given both one-on-one and in group sessions with the patients, the latter much like evangelical revival meetings.

Medication adherence—taking the ARVs on time, all of the time—was the potential Achilles heel of ARV therapy worldwide: if they weren't taken religiously, the efficacy of these drugs would fade, and hope for long-term survival from AIDS would vanish. Indeed, at the Durban conference in 2000, Westerners in attendance quietly wondered whether Africans could be counted on to take their ARVs faithfully, but the doubters were wrong. Like regimental drill sergeants, nurses in Botswana's AIDS clinics would beat into their patients two cardinal precepts: ARV therapy was life-long, and it had to be taken one hundred percent of the time. Failure to do so would bring dishonor on yourself, your family, and your village—indeed, on the entire nation. One of the remarkable aspects of Botswana's HIV Programme was how easily, almost effortlessly, most patients from the start fitted into the medical mold poured for them. Perhaps because the *muti* of traditional healers also had to be taken strictly as directed, the Batswana likewise understood the importance of ARV adherence. God have mercy on anyone who did not take their ARVs like they should: like a scolding mother, the nurse would lecture the disobedient patient.

The patient receiving ARV instruction first thing this morning was a typical case: in his late twenties, he looked much older. His mother was with him and looked much younger than her sick son. He probably had wasted away to almost half his original body weight. A ragged leather belt suspended his baggy black trousers, and on it was stark documentation of the relentless ravages of AIDS: a series of five or six extra buckle holes had been punched into the belt, to accommodate the inexorable shrinkage of his waistline. The patient was also wearing a heavy blue overcoat, and on the floor, next to him, was his walking stick. His black shoes, once formal dress shoes, were worn and scuffed, and had no laces. His mother sat in a chair beside him, carefully listening to the nurse's instructions. He himself, probably because of HIV dementia, seemed less engaged, and needed repeated reminders by the nurse to pay attention.

The nurse was showing the patient and his mother sample tablets of Combivir and efavirenz, as well as printed handouts describing in both English and Setswana the common side effects of the medicines.

Combivir and efavirenz were "first-line" ARVs here, and at the time, were first-line even in the West. I would tell my KITSO classes that a rich HIV-positive New Yorker, going to his private doctor on Fifth Avenue, would be started on the same ARV regimen used as first-line in Botswana. I would boast that first-line therapy here "is not a Toyota Corolla—it's a BMW or Mercedes-Benz!"

Today, the nurse was especially kind and patient. Her instructions to patient and mother sounded like an incantation, as if the soft, melodic cadences of Setswana were calling forth the magical powers of the life-giving ARVs. This seemingly mundane interaction, which was being repeated scores of times across the country that very moment, epitomized the fusion—or collision—of the National ARV Programme with a proud and ancient culture.

I'd now been in Botswana for only six months, and I sensed that it was far too early to discern the full scope of these seismic events. A few foolish people, all from the West and eager to be among the first to report on the medical experiment being undertaken here, had already tried to describe this phenomenon in various articles and news reports. But the real story probably could not be told for at least another ten, maybe even twenty, years. The Batswana were becoming "medicalized." Before, when someone had an ache or pain, the first stop would often be the traditional healer, who would prescribe muti, usually a concoction of herbs. If that failed, the patient would go to the local clinic, usually run by nurses, where the chances of success would probably be no better. Once the symptom resolved, the patient wouldn't return for care until sick again. Except for childhood immunizations and TB treatment—countrywide public health programs which Botswana could be proud of—preventive medicine in Botswana was largely non-existent. But now, with ARVs, patients were told that they would have to return for regular, every-three-month appointments, and would also have to come back to the clinic every month for refills of the ARVs. Previously unknown to most people here, especially the poor and those living in remote villages, a life-long relationship with healthcare services was now expected of them.

The adherence instructions for the patient and his mother were now winding down. It was apparent that the patient, more of an observer than a participant in the teaching, would get better only if his mother gave him the ARVs. The nurse and mother began to chat away in a congenial give-and-take, perhaps about the patient's diet, or how family members were going to help, or maybe about an upcoming church event. Undoubtedly the nurse had also asked the mother if she herself had been HIV tested, as well as whether the patient's partner and children, if any, had also been tested, counselling them to do so if they hadn't already. In America, such questions would have been regarded as "invasive" and a violation of "patient confidentiality," but here they were routine: AIDS was always a family affair.

During all this time, Dr. Moyo had been quietly writing on the patient's outpatient card. Except for hospital inpatient records, there were no centralized medical records in Botswana, and patients carried with them their own outpatient records, a system which accommodated the free flow of medical information in a population which was often mobile and would seek care from clinics in different parts of the country. Standardized in format, these outpatient cards were 8.5 by eleven inches in size, blue for males and pink for females. Infants and children had their own cards, which charted growth and development curves and immunizations. Patients on TB therapy had smaller, separate outpatient cards, on which the clinic would check off every day's dose of anti-TB medicines. On the outpatient cards were written—more often, illegibly scribbled—notes by the doctor or nurse. Medication prescriptions were also written on the cards, and a patient—someone with active TB, for example—could then go to any clinic dispensary in the country to have the prescription filled. Only rarely would a patient forget to bring their outpatient cards for a clinic visit. Most patients carried their cards in cardboard folders or binders, which they would often decorate with pictures of movie stars or colorful scenes cut out from magazines or newspapers. To further customize their out-patient records, many patients would affix little handles on the folder, to make them look like small briefcases. On occasion, as with the patient today, the cards would be stored in a transparent plastic folder, without any personalized decoration.

Dr. Moyo finished his notes, and, without comment, put the cards in the patient's folder and handed them to the mother. This was the signal that the visit was over, and that their next stop would be the pharmacy, to pick up the patient's first supply of ARVs. Haltingly, the patient struggled to stand. Everyone watched passively as he finally made it to his feet on the third try. I reached over and handed him his walking stick. Holding on to his mother's arm, he slowly shuffled to the door. Mother and son had barely cleared the doorway of the consultation room before the next patients in the pressing queue outside pushed into the room.

The patients were a family of five: husband, wife, and their three children, aged four, seven and nine, all HIV-positive. The man, in his early thirties, was a janitor at the hospital. It was somewhat unusual for husbands or fathers to come to the clinic with their infected spouses or children. Too often the men absconded, abandoning wife and children at the first indication any of them had HIV. Of course, these same men, once they learned that they themselves were HIV-positive, usually when they were at death's door, expected their wives or female relatives to look after them.

I quickly handed over my chair to the seven-year-old girl and her nine-year-old brother, who squeezed onto it, directly behind their parents. They were dressed in school uniforms, and although thin, didn't appear to be sickly. Their four-year-old brother looked more malnourished and stood beside his mother, clinging very closely to her, sometimes resting his head in her lap. Except for minimal wasting—no positive "belt buckle sign" here—the father appeared nondescript, and during the entire visit said nothing, appearing annoyed or embarrassed by their situation. The mother was obviously the rock, the long-suffering, fearless source of whatever strength her family needed to prevail. Silently reassuring her fidgety four-year-old at her side, she radiated dignity and quiet confidence. Nobody knew the troubles, the unspoken sorrows she had endured, probably without tears. Inquisitive and wide-eyed, the older brother and sister occasionally turned around to stare at me standing in a corner behind them. Throughout the visit they said nothing, their eyes expressing intelligence and a quiet curiosity. The kids were lucky: too many children had to come to the clinic with their grandmas, aunties, or older sisters, their mothers having died from AIDS, and their fathers having died or being nowhere to be found.

Dr. Moyo explained that several months ago the father had recovered from cryptococcal meningitis, a life-threatening and common complication of AIDS in Botswana. He had initially resisted HIV testing, but finally agreed only after his wife and three children stepped forward and had been tested first. The mother's defiance in deciding to be tested had required great courage: her children's health was paramount, even if it risked abandonment by her husband, whose government job was their only security.

All five of them had been started on ARVs three months previously, and were returning for routine follow-up. Using the mother as spokesperson for the entire family, including her husband, Dr. Moyo quickly ascertained that everyone was doing fine. He then turned the visit over to the nurse, who reviewed with the mother how she was giving the ARVs to the children, and probably her husband as well. The mother had brought along her children's medicines, which were in separate paper bags, each with the child's name on it. With proud efficiency, she demonstrated to the nurse the various doses she had been giving to her children—for such young patients, the ARVs had to be individually dosed according to weight and height. Except for a few minor clarifications, the nurse was satisfied, and then went on to ask about the adults' ARV regimens. The mother spoke for both herself and her husband, again reassuring the nurse that there were no problems taking the medicines as directed. Her husband remained passive, giving only grudging, mute nods to the nurse's questions. This was the last place he wanted to be. The only part of the visit remaining was drawing blood tests from everyone, to be sure the ARVs were working. On their way out—the seven- and nine-year-olds were probably going on to school—the older boy looked back at me, and, serious and unsmiling, waved goodbye.

There was a brief delay in the arrival of the next patient. He was a 32-year-old prisoner, slowly carried into the room by another pris- oner, both dressed in standard orange jumpsuits. The patient was almost gone, practically skeletal. His compatriot gently cradled him onto the exam table. Glassy-eyed through deep bony sockets, the patient gave out a soft moan as the bones of his bottom touched the hard mat on the table. The other prisoner tried to reposition him, to lessen his discomfort, looking down on him with profound worry and concern. Following at a safe distance was their guard, young and striking in his crisp uniform, black boots, wide black belt, and epaulettes, all highly polished. Appearing annoyed to be here, he brusquely dismissed his helper, who looked as if he wished he could stay and look after his fellow inmate. I gazed dumbly at the scene before me. What was the connection between these two guys, other than being prisoners? Friends, relatives, lovers, or perhaps just two people who cared about each other, when no one else did?

Dr. Moyo thumbed through the sparse records sent from the prison. Medical care in the prisons here was as bad as that in Ameri- can prisons early-on in the epidemic. His T-cell count a year ago was three, and he'd been having protracted vomiting and diarrhea. He had never been started on ARVs. As Moyo quickly examined him, the guard stood in a corner, as far away as possible, arms pro- tectively folded over his chest. His nervous gaze never wavered from his charge—it encompassed disgust, aversion, and fear. I didn't have to wonder whether he'd ever been HIV tested.

Moyo quickly concluded that the patient needed hospitaliza- tion for intravenous fluids for dehydration. I concurred, but added that there was no way he could take his ARVs on his own in the hospital. For reasons I never understood, nurses in government hospitals were not permitted to administer them to inpatients, and either the patient or family members had to be responsible for storing and taking them. If the patient was confused or demented and didn't have family that visited daily, he was out of luck. I turned and asked the guard if the patient had any family nearby. Embarrassed and annoyed at being included in anything to do with the plague, he tersely replied that "maybe" the prisoner's home village was in Gweta, hundreds of miles away. Unlike the previous patients seen that day, the prisoner was probably doomed: it was unlikely he would make it out of hospital alive, for another chance at being started on ARVs. Moyo scribbled a few notes in the patient's record, and then put him on IV fluids. Summoned back, the other prisoner re-entered and carried the patient out to the medical ward. Exiting, the guard averted his eyes from me.

The procession of patients continued. Younger patients were accompanied by older family members—mothers, grandmothers, great-grandmothers, aunts, older sisters. Older patients, many in their seventies and eighties, would be accompanied by their children, grandchildren, or younger siblings. As usual, there were scant males as supportive partners or family members. AIDS often blurred generational differences, rendering chronological age irrelevant. A thirty-three-year-old woman, who weighed less than half of her baseline body weight, looked simultaneously very old and very young, like one of those unfortunate children with rare genetic defects causing them to age prematurely. Sex among the very old was never regarded as unusual here, so no one was surprised when someone in his nineties had HIV. Indeed, as the nurses had assured me earlier, here a man became old only when he died.

The informal sense of "family" in the Molepolole clinic could become a bit too loose. Rarely was any patient visit not interrupted at least once by someone walking into the consultation room, always without knocking. A nurse would need a lab form or some blood collection tubes. A patient seen earlier in the day might have forgotten to ask for a medication refill, or to tell the doctor about a symptom, which the doctor would take care of in front of the patient already in the room. A housekeeper would have to empty the trash from the previous day. A nurse from an inpatient ward would walk in to tell the doctor about a patient problem. The doctors in the ARV clinics also had inpatient duties as well, and often had to leave the clinic to assist a midwife with a complicated delivery, or to pronounce a patient dead, in order to free up a bed for one of the other patients lying on floor mattresses or on a gurney in the hallway. These interruptions were part of the natural rhythm of all of the clinics here, and no one thought much about them.

The parade of patients continued, unabated.

A seventeen-year-old girl was next in line for ARV initiation. Obese and dressed in a threadbare halter dress and tatty tennis shoes, she appeared emotionless and uninterested, and was totally oblivious of being well into the third trimester of pregnancy. It was obvious she was definitely with child. Accompanying her was her equally heavy mother, who likewise professed no clue about the obvious protrusion of her daughter's tummy. "This girl, she is retarded," volunteered the nurse, more with resignation than anything else. Blank looks from patient and mother. When Dr. Moyo questioned the patient about the pregnancy, she replied that there was "a growth down there," pointing to her vagina. He was able to hear a strong fetal heartbeat, and let the patient listen with his stethoscope. She appeared intrigued. Determined not to be left out, the mother slowly hoisted herself out of the chair, elbowed her way to the exam table, and listened for herself.

Simple enough: another pregnant HIV mother, albeit a bit slow-witted. There's a national protocol for that—PMTCT, prevention of mother-to-child transmission. But things here are never easy: extensive vaginal warts protruded from her vagina, moist cauliflower-like lesions, blocking the vaginal opening. The girl's vaginal warts were serious enough to merit an eventual Caesarean section. ARVs were started, but she was also referred to the PMTCT Programme. Moyo would see her in two weeks, when he would also schedule her for a C-section. Shaking her head in dismay, the nurse added to her usual adherence lecture a discussion of the facts of life.

"She doesn't know who the father is, but I think I do," the nurse observed dryly. "I know the mother," she added, nodding in her direction with no attempt to conceal her disgust. "She's no help. Her church preaches against condoms. They also practice enemas for spiritual cleansing, and they use the same tube for everyone. We have a big problem with these people." I had heard about such practices, which, hygiene aside, could transmit HIV. As they left the room, mother and mother-to-be seemed happy with the attention given to them, and were smiling broadly.

Next was a twenty-four-year-old man from a nearby village, here to start ARVs, but he hadn't brought along an adherence partner. At this early moment in Botswana's Treatment Programme, every-one—above all, the nurses— looked askance at starting someone on ARVs without a friend, partner, or family member to help them take their medicines. Normally, I would have been sympathetic to such a patient, since disclosure of one's HIV status was sometimes too great a leap to take. But there was a grating arrogance in this guy's man-ner, which came to the fore when, despite repeated prodding from the nurse, he adamantly refused to notify his former girlfriend to get tested. He had every possible excuse, every one self-serving: that she would blame him if she tested positive, that if she tested positive she could have got it from someone else, that she could have given it to him, that he was too busy, and so on. The more he talked, the less I liked him. "This jerk's probably like those morons on the roads who risk not only their own lives, but everyone else's," I thought to myself as I sat back and observed the gathering storm.

No amount of counseling and coercion from the nurse could cause him to act with decency, to stop blaming others for his situation. As their conversation switched from English to Setswana, it became louder and heated. The nurse finally gave up. "*This one,*" she said, glaring at the patient with contempt, "this one is a problem. He won't tell his partner who moved to the next village. And since she left, he now has sex with young girls in his village and won't use protection. I think he's the father of the baby with that young retarded girl who didn't know she was pregnant. They are neighbors, and he takes care of their goats." It was scary: the nurses here knew *everything.* "Yes, this one is a big problem. And he says he knows his rights and will go to the minister if he is not started on ARVs." The nurse sat back in her chair, disapprovingly folding her arms on her chest, seething at the patient through squinting eyes.

The patient looked passively ahead, but with a tinge of arrogance that provoked the nurse to violently jerk around her chair so that her back was now to him. Moyo turned to me for advice. Time for me to be professional and overlook the fact the patient was a jerk.

"The national guidelines do not absolutely require an adherence partner to be present," I replied very slowly. The last thing I wanted to do was to undermine the nurse, whose pride had already been grievously injured. "If we feel the patient understands his medication regimen, we are obliged to start it. Moreover"—and here I spoke directly to the nurse—"it's better to get him on ARVs, to decrease his chances of infecting others. It's the lesser of two evils, sister." I practically pleaded with her, as if she had the ultimate say over whether we started him on ARVs.

"Do we refuse to start him on ARVs because he's not a nice person and does bad things, and thus let him continue to infect people, or do we accept the fact that he's a bad person and protect the village by starting him on ARVs? If he's on ARVs, he's much less likely to infect anyone. 'Blessed are the merciful,' right, sister?" The appeal by way of the Beatitudes did the trick: the nurse sullenly turned her chair around towards the patient, and, without looking at him directly, coldly instructed him on how to take his ARVs.

Yes, a lesser of two evils: I had indirectly given him permission to have sex without condoms, which he would do anyway. But the ARVs would hopefully protect his partners from HIV, though not pregnancy and other sexually transmitted diseases. In medicine, it is called risk reduction. Quietly gloating, the man left the consultation room with his ARV prescription.

"Thank you, sister. You really made the right decision. You've probably saved quite a few people from infection." Her smile assured me that I hadn't pissed her off.

Even at this early moment in my stay in Botswana, I tried to be philosophical: it was, after all, *their* AIDS crisis, not mine. You had to disavow the grand plans of WHO, the CDC, UNAIDS, and the myriad other alphabet agencies from the West, which were falling all over each other in Botswana. Their emphasis on targeting large numbers of people—plans which had yet to bear any fruit—seemed at times to evoke Stalin's remark that the loss of a single life was a great tragedy, whereas the loss of a million lives was a mere statistic. Here, snatching just one person from the jaws of AIDS was a miracle, and "saving" tens of thousands was just a statistic, mere pie in the sky. "One life at a time" made more sense to me, and helped me put my role here into better perspective.

A bit after 11 a.m., it was teatime, and everything stopped. It was a countrywide ritual, a silly holdover from the Brits, especially since there were still lots of patients waiting to be seen. In many clinics, the nurses would take their tea and biscuits at the nursing station, in full view of patients, many of whom, having left before dawn, hadn't eaten for many hours. I politely declined Dr. Moyo's invitation to join them in the medical staffroom. I stretched out my legs and relished the solitude. The consult room was in the back of the prefab building, and its window opened onto bush. The curtains lazily flapped in the warm breeze. Several cows were grazing right outside, their neck bells tinkling gently. I leaned back, closed my eyes, and once again relished the time and space of Botswana.

After tea, the procession of patients continued.

There was a thirty-six-year-old woman, coming to commence ARV therapy, accompanied by her twin brother, who was to be her adherence partner. Dressed in a grey overcoat, matching bright-orange dress and head-dress, and worn tennis shoes, she appeared fairly generic: moderately malnourished, but not yet a walking skeleton. She still had hope of rescue. Her brother, the supposed adherence partner, was much weaker and slower, and struggled with his cane to ease into his chair. His baggy brown pants, probably once suit pants, were suspended around his wisp of a waistline by a faded yellow necktie, strung through the belt loops and knotted in front. The tie design was a panoply of smiling teddy bears. Moyo didn't pay the brother much attention, but the nurse was staring at him uneasily, gently rocking back and forth in her chair, arms folded across her chest. The man sensed her scrutiny, and fixed his gaze onto the floor.

As soon as Moyo finished his interview of the woman, the nurse launched into an animated interrogation of the brother in Setswana. Her tone was like that of a worried mother with a wayward child, both critical and concerned. Head bent downwards, the man appeared ashamed, and responded to her queries with only a shaking of his head in the negative. But the nurse did not give up, and in equal measure she pleaded, cajoled, berated, and lectured the man. His sister also chimed in, and it was apparent that she, too, was worried about her brother. The man did not alter his downward gaze. It was a matter which could not be surmounted. After nearly five minutes, the nurse stopped, and turned to Moyo and me.

"This one," she gestured with frustration, "this one has been sick for a long time, but he refuses to be tested. His wife died here last year, and his youngest child died last month. The nurses have tried to convince him, but he refuses. His sister has tried, but he refuses. Their mother died two months ago, and their father left her for a younger woman when she got sick, but he still refuses. They only have each other. He used to be a teacher, but now stays at home all day." Then, with a shrug of resignation, "What are we to do?" I sympathetically shrugged and shook my head in agreement. Nothing could be done. He was one of those who would go to his grave rather than be HIV tested.

The nurse focused now on the sister and in short order reviewed the ARVs with her. The sister seemed well prepared, and the interaction with the nurse was warm and cordial. It was assumed that the brother, her "adherence partner," would be of no help, so he was left out of the conversation. As the sister left, she had to help her brother get up from the chair. Arm in arm, they exited, the brother never once looking up.

By early afternoon, the clinic was winding down. The other doctors would have to see the remaining patients, because Moyo wanted me to see two of his patients in the hospital. As we walked to the medical ward, he briefed me on the first one. Matilda had been the head nurse of the HIV clinic from its opening, where she worked right up to the time when she was admitted for cryptococcal meningitis.

"Last week this time, she was sitting at the clinic entrance, checking blood pressures and weights. She was very weak, and couldn't walk. The other nurses helped her get around. Her husband died from HIV a few months back. Her last day or so, she couldn't even check blood pressures, and she just sat there and directed the patients."

"Was she taking ARVs?" I thought it was a fair question.

"Oh, she never got tested," Moyo replied, a bit embarrassed.

"I never asked her. I think one of the other nurses might have talked to her about it. I don't know." Although healthcare workers regularly asked—*demanded*—that patients get tested, they often refused to be tested themselves. And I'm sure Matilda also exhorted people to be tested. But not herself. I really couldn't get on my high horse about it: I myself hadn't been tested for almost a year, and I wasn't a monk.

The adult medical ward was full of patients, but was quiet—not in a sepulchral way, just peaceful and calm. Unlike the States, there were no armies of nurses bustling about with their medication carts, no technicians taking ECGs or drawing blood, no escorts ferrying patients to physical therapy or for MRI scans. No, here it was unhurried. Each of the three large rooms in the ward had eight beds, rusted and ancient, plus a half-dozen or so mattresses on the floor, between the beds, for the overflow of additional patients. Rickety tray tables and bedside stands were cluttered with food and juices brought in by relatives. The rooms were clean, and the place reflected more a lack of resources than the depressing squalor of my AIDS ward in New York City ten years earlier.

A few patients were lying or sitting in their beds, while others lounged on tattered sofa chairs in the hallway, watching a South African soap opera on an old TV securely fastened to the wall. A few of the nurses and housekeeping staff were also watching TV. Some patients indeed looked thin and malnourished—and a few beds were occupied with motionless, skeletal specters—but many patients appeared reasonably well. On my AIDS ward in New York in the early 1990s, there had always been an all-pervasive gloom and despair. At that bleak time in the epidemic, most of my patients—the homeless, drug addicts, prisoners—had been pariahs long before AIDS arrived. But for almost all of the patients at Scottish Livingstone, AIDS had interrupted largely full and happy lives. The patients here could very likely be neighbors, friends, or even relatives, but not outcasts. Molepolole's medical ward was suffused with neither gloom nor joy. Rather, an air of inertia seemed to hover over it, and the antique ceiling fans slowly wobbling overhead were making the only noticeable perturbation to the state of things.

Moyo led me to the female room. Matilda was lying on her back in bed, dead. If it was possible, she looked more wasted than the worst patient I had seen there so far. Her dark-blue nursing cloak covered her from the waist down. Pinned on a lapel of the cloak, along with her nursing school pin, was a red AIDS ribbon. I recalled a very similar dark blue nursing cloak that my mother wore to work sixty years previously in Ohio. The other patients in the ward seemed unaware of Matilda's departure. I reached over and closed her eyes.

Moyo scribbled a brief death note on Matilda's chart, and as we moved on to his next patient in the male ward, he told me his story. Thapelo—Setswana for "prayer"—was a twenty-four-year-old student at the University of Botswana, and had been admitted a week previously for pneumonia, which had been worsening in spite of antibiotics. Thapelo also had KS, and the characteristic purplish spots on his face and lower legs had been enlarging and spreading over the past week. Because he had repeatedly refused HIV testing, Moyo went ahead and obtained a T-cell count instead, which was fifty-six. Even when confronted with this evidence of severe immune suppression, Thapelo still refused HIV testing, which was necessary before he could be started on ARVs. Earlier today, Thapelo's breathing had become more labored. Moyo was very worried.

At the bedside, I saw that Thapelo was on his way out. He was propped up in bed, his respirations shallow and rapid. Small beads of perspiration coated his forehead, and a drop of sweat was dangling on the tip of his nose, which was encrusted with a dark-purple lesion. Even with the blotches of KS over his face, Thapelo was a handsome young man, and he weakly smiled a greeting to us. He tried to speak, but his lungs wouldn't let him. As I listened to his chest, I admired his massively broad and muscular shoulders. That was the scary thing about AIDS: you didn't have to be a skeleton in order to have an immune system shot to hell. Thapelo's back and chest were clammy and moist from perspiration, and his breath sounds were wet and crackly. I wiped the sweat on my stethoscope onto his sheets. The nurse had brought his chest X-ray to the bedside. I squinted at it through the sunlight from the adjacent window—there was no X-ray view box—and it looked terrible: diffuse pneumonia, almost a total "white-out" of both lungs. I turned back to Thapelo and held his hand, stroking it with my thumb.

"I'm very worried, Thapelo," I said in a deliberate, subdued tone, trying to balance concern with reassurance. "You have a very bad pneumonia. It could be due to TB, PCP—the AIDS pneumonia—or your KS, or all three." Struggling for air, Thapelo nodded understanding. "I think we have to treat you for all these possibilities." Raising the subject of HIV testing yet again could frighten him further. "Hang in there. We're also going to start you on some morphine, to decrease your discomfort. It will help you rest." Almost as an involuntary reflex, I gently squeezed his hand, and he squeezed back, ever so weakly and briefly. A mixture of sadness and longing washed over me, welcome proof that the sea of need around me hadn't drowned my ability to care. It was more and more difficult for me to mourn without being overwhelmed by the unending suffering everywhere. But the alternative—not to be moved by what was before me—would be even more disquieting. I briefly thought back to Matilda and the sight of her lying there covered by her nursing cloak, a shroud that had brought back memories of my own mother's career.

Out in the hallway, I discussed Thapelo's case with Moyo. Seat-of-the-pants "shot gun" therapy was his only hope, and chemotherapy for KS and antibiotic therapy for TB, PCP, and bacterial pneumonia were in order. TB, PCP, and bacterial pneumonia—these Moyo could treat at Scottish. But chemotherapy for the KS would have to be ordered from Gaborone, a process that could take several weeks. Transferring Thapelo to Marina would be too risky—besides, it would take days for the oncologists there to see him and start the chemo, even if they could be persuaded to do so. I did suggest putting him on oxygen, but Moyo said that all of the hospital's oxygen tanks were empty. The next shipment wouldn't arrive until the next week at the earliest.

I concluded with one of the last rites in medicine. "You need to start him on 'round-the-clock morphine," I said as I was writing a brief note in the chart. "He's a big guy, so I'd start at 10mg and titrate upwards as needed. I'd be sure he gets it every four hours, straight order, unless he's sleeping." In addition to reducing pain, morphine would also relieve Thapelo's discomfort—and fear— from his breathlessness. "Ten, 15, even 20mg isn't going to knock his lights out, but it might ease his transition."

"It's a shame really," Moyo observed. "My wife knows the family. He was a top student, very serious, and he was working on his thesis with Professor Kenneth Good, before the controversy set in." Everyone in Botswana knew about the much-celebrated Professor Good brouhaha, which the local newspapers had been covering with daily front-page articles.

Thapelo's connection with Professor Good indicated a mind interested in ideas and current events, and not just with getting drunk every night, as many students did. A teacher at the University of Botswana, Professor Good had recently been declared a "PI"— prohibited immigrant—and the government had ordered him deported from the country. Although the case was being reviewed as an urgent petition to the High Court, it was a hopeless challenge: Botswana's Constitution gave the President the right to declare anyone a PI, without having to give any justification. Even naturalized citizens could be deported without cause, and Good, an expatriate from Australia, was not even a citizen. According to the press, Good's transgression had been his increasing attacks on the succession provisions of the Constitution, which in effect guaranteed that the Vice-President would automatically succeed the President. There were many people in Botswana, Good among them, who did not want Vice-President Ian Khama to become President someday.

Yet in Botswana, controversies such as this one were often not what they seemed. The political elite here did not feel threatened by the strong views of an old man like Good. He had not incited people to riot, and the students were not up in arms. And President Mogae was an extremely tolerant man with a very thick skin, not given to pettiness. Rather, Good had been collaborating with Survival International, a London-based advocacy group for indigenous peoples. For years, this organization had denounced Botswana for its proposed resettlement of the San, an aboriginal race, from the central Kalahari Desert to other locations in the country because, so it was claimed, the reserve they occupied was rich in diamonds. To dramatize its case, Survival International had been portraying Botswana's precious stones and the source of its new-found wealth as "blood diamonds," a term the international community used to describe the diamonds which financed bloody civil wars in other African countries, especially Liberia and Sierra Leone. Diamonds were Botswana's lifeline, and had allowed the country a standard of living higher than that of other African countries. Its hospitals and clinics, its universal education system which taught even the poorest citizens how to read and write English, the ARV Programme itself—all of this was made possible by the diamond mines in the country. Mess with Botswana's diamonds, and you're meddling with primal forces.

Thapelo's past political activism at the university also exemplified how AIDS had been a godsend to the political and financial elite of Botswana, as in other areas of the continent. AIDS had created a social stasis, a comfortable inertia for the elites, since everyone was preoccupied with surviving the plague. Disparities of wealth could be attributed to AIDS, and not the political system. Many potential revolutionaries, or intellectuals who might challenge the status quo, were dying. But because of ARVs, other Thapelos would live to challenge the status quo.

On the mid-afternoon drive back to Gaborone, I reviewed in my mind the patients I'd seen earlier. I was satisfied we did the best we could. Mostly, I thought about Thapelo and his struggle to die, a struggle all of us would one day face. Over my many years as a doctor, I'd seen many Thapelos and witnessed their struggles, their transitions from life. I'd come to realize that it's one thing to contemplate your eventual mortality from the safe remove of good health and a relatively young age. It's quite another thing to go through it yourself. I vowed to remember Thapelo when it was my turn.

My journey back to Gaborone was a bit less solitary than my morning drive: my "friends," the mid-afternoon clouds, had arrived. Their silent advent always lifted my spirits, filling the glaring void of the morning sky. As the two-lane road became a modern four-lane highway on the capital's outskirts, I felt mildly exhilarated that I was back in "civilization." Future outreach trips made me appreciate Gaborone, so ground down were most of the places I'd visit. After a trip to Kasane, Molepolole, or—worse—Hukuntsi, Ghanzi, or Tshabong, I understood how Gaborone, for the Batswana at least, was the big city.

Later, at dusk, I sat alone on my porch, still thinking about the patients I'd seen earlier in the day. The sun had just set, and a new moon was about to take over the heavens. The distant thunderclouds had almost dissolved into the pinkish ether and were now flat, slate-grey outlines against the darkening blue sky. I felt very, very alone. Gazing blankly at my walled-in yard, I focused on a small weaver bird hopping through the leaves and brown grass. It was scouring the ground for just the right twig for its nest, then flying off with it and disappearing into a nearby tree. A minute or so later, the bird returned, and resumed scavenging for another twig, and so on, with almost rhythmic regularity. Some twigs were too big, others too small. But the bird was patient and industrious in its instinctual ritual of nest building. I felt connected to the world again.

From another tree the hooting of a solitary red-eyed dove echoed through the gathering darkness. I recalled my very first evening here many months earlier, after a long flight from the States to a new job in a new and strange continent. I had been sitting out on the same porch, crazed by jet lag and wondering what I was doing here, so far from friends and family. That's when I first heard the red-eyed dove's plaintive call. Back then, it sounded foreign, cautionary, as if to announce an ancient premonition. Yes, that first night in Botswana, the dove seemed to be warning, "Take heed. You are now in Africa."

The deep cooing finally stopped, and the only sound was the distant traffic. I wondered if Thapelo was still alive. It was now dark.

# Chapter 8

## Local Flora and Fauna: "Are You or Have You Ever Been an Imbecile?"

There it was, listed among the otherwise routine questions on the application for my Botswana driver's license: "Are you or have you ever been an imbecile?" By this point in early 2003, in the country for four months, I was already accustomed to the singular idiosyncrasies—the wackiness—that could pop up anytime and anywhere. When I later asked the clerk handing me my new license how long it was good for, her answer likewise didn't surprise me: "Why, *it's good for life!*" the smiling young woman said breathlessly, seeming to take delight in her reply. It was the Batswana's genuine zest for living in the moment that leavened the sad stories I encountered daily.

The surest way to realize, as Dorothy said in *The Wizard of Oz*, you weren't in Kansas anymore was to read the local newspapers. There were at least a half-dozen daily papers in Botswana, plus a couple of weekly ones. The stories in the dailies ranged from the semi-serious to the seriously deranged, and provided insight into everyday life there. America's *National Enquirer* and similar tabloids had nothing on the ones in Botswana.

Probably my all-time favorite newspaper headline was "City Police Arrest Serial Donkey Rapist." The article itself didn't give many details about the alleged perpetrator of such outrage, except that he was transferred to the Mental Hospital thirty miles to the south. Wild donkeys were everywhere in Botswana, and most people never paid them any mind, unless, as often happened, they'd saunter across a busy highway or, especially irksome, would choose to just stand in the middle of the road, clogging up traffic even more than usual. A close second in the Bizarre Newspaper Articles Hall of Fame, at least for me, was an article—an expose—revealing that female prisoners working in the kitchen at the main prison had been secreting away large carrots and English cucumbers, grown in the prison's garden, for use as sex toys, "pleasuring themselves," as the article salaciously reported. This scandalous story might never have made the light of day if one of the kitchen workers hadn't refused to share her vegetables with her cellmate.

As everywhere else in the world, sex was the prime subject in the tabloids. Stories of jealous lovers hacking up their rivals and feeding them to the dogs were a dime a dozen. One article reported on the controversy about whether male prisoners should have access to condoms, since acknowledgement of same-sex activity behind bars was anathema to the prison governor, who fulminated against such "immoral and indecent behavior." The writer had interviewed a former prisoner, who, anonymously, reported that such illicit sexual activity was not unusual in the prisons. "And before he knew it," the article continued about this eyewitness, "after entering prison he was soon touching his toes to accommodate the impure needs of his prison mates." The official statute prohibiting homosexual liaisons in Botswana defined "sodidodimy"—yes, that's the word the statute and newspapers used—as "carnal knowledge of one's anus," certainly a mind-twisting definition.

An ongoing saga in the papers, one which was still going on over ten years after it first hit the news, was the Daisy Loo fiasco.

It's one of those incredible stories that has been clogging up the courts for over a decade and has provided much employment to the lawyers. Probably no one, not even the legions of lawyers and judges involved in the case, could describe its circuitous evolution accurately. In a nutshell, around 2005 the Gaborone City Council (GCC), the municipal government for the capital, asked for bids to cut grass and clear brush in a largely abandoned area in the city. Daisy Loo Cleaning Company put in a bid for twenty-one million pula, then between two and three million dollars. Now, this bid was extraordinary, since the area to be cleared was small and the job itself might take a day or so to complete—imagine asking millions of dollars just to mow one of the several lawns in Central Park. But even more remarkable was that someone in the GCC accepted the bid and signed a contract with Daisy Loo. The job was quickly done according to the specifications. When Daisy Loo tried to collect, the GCC balked, and the company got a court judgment in its favor, which the GCC ignored. When a deputy sheriff, an officer of the court, started to enforce the court ruling by carting up and removing furniture, vans, cars, TVs, and computers from the expansive GCC offices, someone in the GCC issued Daisy Loo a check for 21,434,434.46 pula, a princely sum that could otherwise pay for filling all the potholes in the city for many years to come. But before Daisy Loo could cash it, the government agency responsible for ferreting out corruption had payment stopped. Ever since then, the case has been wending its way through the courts, with some people accused of collusion and corruption. Now, to be fair, you would have to devote your entire life to this case to understand it, but the overall story is quite simple: a cleaning company and the GCC agreed to a fee of twenty-one million to do a minor job of cleaning and cutting brush.

The more serious newspapers did cover politics, but the machinations of the many political parties gave new meaning to the words "arcane" and "byzantine." The Botswana Democratic Party had such a lock-hold on power that the petty political maneuverings seemed inconsequential. However, a few of the papers would challenge the government, and after Ian Khama became Vice-President in 1998, they relentlessly pounded away at his alleged penchant for spying and domestic surveillance, especially electronic eavesdropping. Indeed, the press would regularly pillory and berate the antics and schemes of the rich and powerful in Botswana—for reasons I could never understand, they were called "big shorts," not big shots—but always to no avail. The *Sunday Standard*—often dubbed the "Sunday Substandard"—had weekly front-page stories about alleged malfeasance by government officials and prominent businessmen, the sort of stuff that in the States would result in grand jury indictments and special prosecutors. But after several weeks of running variations on the same story, the paper would latch onto another apparent scandal, while the presumed perpetrators of the prior brouhaha drifted into obscurity. Time was always on the side of the rich and powerful.

A perennial target of the *Sunday Standard* was the head of the shadowy Directorate of Intelligence Services (DIS), Botswana's FBI and CIA combined, an agency that seemed accountable to no one, including the President. The allegations were mind-boggling— imagine the head of the FBI accepting gifts of stock from a company the FBI was actively investigating—but DIS was immune. J. Edgar Hoover was a shrinking violet compared with the leader of DIS, who was probably more powerful and feared than Ian Khama. The irony was that the head of DIS had formerly been Ian's "batman," or personal valet, when he was at university in the UK. Ian later made him an integral part of the nation's intelligence services.

Sometimes there were stories that were part of the folklore, and you didn't know whether to believe them or not, although they had a ring of Botswana truth to them. According to one of them from many years ago, an Appeals Court judge, outfitted in crimson judicial robes and white full-bottomed wig, let off a rapist caught in the act by piously opining, "A woman's open legs are a flowing river every man must cross." There were audible gasps in the courtroom as people looked around and asked, "Did he just say what I thought he said?" The judge, who had been imported from a West African country, was soon thereafter kicked out of the country. There were rumors that after he left, they found stashed under his bed, unopened, the copious legal briefs of cases that had been languishing on his docket for over two years.

Botswana is a very religious country. At all of the government ministries, the workday would always start with group prayer and hymns, and every ministry meeting began with prayer. Profanity was deeply censured, and could even result in arrest—I had to watch my language. The Catholic and Anglican cathedrals and the city's main mosque were clustered next to the downtown mall. Scattered throughout the outlying residential areas were innumerable evangelical and Pentecostal churches—the so-called "happy-clappy" churches—where many preachers told their flocks to throw out their ARVs and rely upon prayer for a miracle. "Have any of these pastors stopped to think," I would gently remark at the KITSO courses, "that maybe—just maybe—the ARVs are an answer to all of their prayers for deliverance from AIDS?" My students would always nod in agreement. To gauge a patient's readiness for starting ARVs, I usually asked what his church said about these drugs— sometimes the patient would say his church was against them, but that he still wanted to start. Every so often, a local charlatan would make headlines, as when a Zimbabwean holy roller exhorted his flock to bring in their ARVs and trust everything to the Lord. He then turned around and sold them on the black market back home in Zim, allowing him a lavish lifestyle, with fancy cars and loose women. He was eventually shown the door.

One of the things I wasn't prepared for when I moved to Botswana was the driving. It was a miracle that I never had even a minor fender-bender. The traffic fatality rate in Botswana was twice that of the States. Many drivers just couldn't help themselves whenever they approached an amber traffic light: as if possessed by demons, they would maniacally speed through the intersection three or four seconds *after* the light turned red. And when they stopped at a traffic light, they would slowly nose their cars into the intersection, intent on entering it a millisecond after the light turned green, never mind that another driver on the crossroad might try to speed through several seconds after the light changed. Throughout the city, intersections were carpeted with innumerable, diamond-sized fragments of recently shattered car windows and headlights, remnants of recent crashes. The last Friday of the month—"end-of-month payday"— was especially perilous, as alcohol, speed, and hormones inevitably led to major crashes.

The mayhem of the roads in Botswana was further complicated by the fact that they also belonged to four-legged creatures: herds of goats, their young in tow, frolicking helter-skelter, sometimes overturning roadside trash bins and scattering the detritus onto the road; herds of cows lazily crossing the roads, their herd boys nowhere to be found; and the dumb donkeys standing statue-like in the middle of the road, or like ancient sentinels at the edge of the road, threatening to lurch into the traffic. One afternoon, at the height of rush hour, a large brewery truck overturned on the Western Bypass, a major artery skirting the edge of Gaborone. It was the result of a run-in with a couple of donkeys straying onto the highway. Although no one was hurt, save for the two donkeys, the truck's cargo of Castle beer had not been so lucky: people from a nearby shopping mall and housing settlement clustered onto the highway, carrying away the hundreds of cases of brew strewn around the wreck. Drivers on the highway pulled off to the side of the road, likewise to load up on the largesse. Police called to the scene had also jumped into the melee, helping themselves to the liquid manna from heaven. The newspaper article, which had a half-page photo of the free-for-all, made no mention of any official police explanation for the misconduct. Order finally prevailed when military police from the Botswana Defense Force arrived—they knew that if they, too, helped themselves to the booty, their sorry hides would be caned, since President Ian Khama was a strict teetotaler.

Although the elites looked after themselves, there was still opportunity for even the poorest to move up the social ladder. In my own experience, two of the lowest—a friend's domestic worker and a janitor at another friend's storage business—had sons in the medical school. Public education meant that almost everyone spoke and read English, except possibly some of the San in the Kalahari.

Most Batswana had a devoted love of country, a pride in who they were. Whenever they sang the national anthem, a simple and gentle plaint, not at all bombastic, they did so lovingly. In Botswana "the nation" was part of the fabric of family and village. A few years into the National Programme, to get more people tested and on treatment, the government announced that HIV testing would be an "opt-out" affair: the doctor would say he was getting an HIV test on you, and if you didn't object—opt out—you'd get tested. No intrusive and frightening pre-test counselling. After the initiative was announced through all of the major media in the country, the Batswana swamped the testing stations, out of a sense of national duty, of patriotism. Back then, opt-out testing was a radical step, frowned upon by politically correct AIDS activists in the West, who resisted anything that might weaken HIV exceptionalism. At an international HIV conference soon after Botswana's announcement, several speakers from the West criticized the move as a violation of human rights, as if the government was rounding up people to be forcibly tested against their will. Dr. Ndwapi calmly punctured their self-righteousness by replying, "It works for us." A few years later, the United States government adopted the same policy.

Yes, the Batswana were very much their own people, in both endearing and frustrating ways, often at the same time. Their social IQ was infinitely greater than that of us outsiders—forget ever trying to outsmart them. Even if a situation is hopeless, they will never let on that it is, not out of deviousness but because they don't want to disappoint you. In meetings, their voices are soft, almost inaudible, but in the locker room the decibels are deafening. I'd always tell newcomers that in Botswana, *it's always something*: an important document or application is rejected by a government clerk because it's printed on the wrong-sized paper, never mind we're talking a few millimeters' difference; the internet goes off right before you were about to send a crucial email; the ATM machines are on the blink, again; you can't renew your medical license because the government computers have been down for several weeks.

But at the end of the day, as the sun would sink with blazing majesty and the distant thunderclouds reflected the pinkish glow of the sunset, with the red-eyed dove gently serenading the dusk, all these annoyances evaporated. Although I missed friends and family in the States, there were so many times I really didn't want to be anywhere else in the world.

# Chapter 9

# Holy Cross Hospice

Debra, one of the Hospice nurses, slowly guided the gaunt, hollow-faced woman into the consultation room. She appeared middle-aged, with matted, straggly hair, although she looked like she had aged prematurely. Shoeless and clad in a very thin pink sundress, she was absent-mindedly cradling her baby girl in her left arm. The baby, definitely under one year, was dressed only in a small stained T-shirt on which was a faded picture of the Magic Kingdom at Disney World. Steadying herself with her right hand on the edge of my desk, the woman stood stiffly and wobbled briefly before slowly lowering herself and her baby into the chair. No sentience seemed to emanate from her sunken orbits, and she paid no mind to Debra, me, her baby, or her surroundings. In addition to having no shoes—even the poorest Batswana had shoes—there was another unusual thing about her: she was sobbing quietly. It was rare for even the most desperate, most pathetic patients to cry, their tears having long ago dried up. Tears were usually reserved for the mourners at graveside vigils. The woman looked at the floor, sniffing back tears and wiping them with her free hand. I handed her my nicely ironed white handkerchief. "It's clean," I assured her, as if that made any difference whatsoever.

The baby, aroused from its infant dreams, started to squirm, but the woman ignored her, clutching my handkerchief in her bony hand, but not wiping the small rivulets of tears coursing down both cheeks. The baby started to scream and flail about, but the woman still ignored her, holding her even further away. Debra picked the baby up and gently rocked her back to sleep. The patient had no medical cards. In fact, she had nothing on her other than her flimsy clothing and her baby.

"We found her lying in an alley on home visits to Old Naledi this morning," Debra reported. My nurse had seen similarly sad cases before, so I wasn't surprised at her matter-of-fact tone.

Unlike Puso, the other Hospice "nurse," Debra was a proper nurse, a recent graduate, who was waiting for a job opening at Marina. She lived with her mother in Mochudi, a small village north of Gaborone. Attractive and older than most new graduates, she had a calm, mature aura, and I felt very comfortable around her. Like most Batswana, she was also religious. A few months earlier, Gaborone was in the grip of a drought, while in Mochudi there were downpours. I joked with Debra how unfair it was that she had rain at home, while we city folk were suffering. "Maybe," she said with a smile, "people don't pray enough in Gaborone."

"Neighbors say she's from Gabane," Debra continued. Gabane was a rural community just a few miles outside Gaborone. "She said she lives with a ten-year-old cousin in Old Naledi, but we couldn't find her. She drinks a lot, and leaves the baby with the cousin when she goes out. Her partner in Gabane threw her out. She said her partner put a curse on her."

The woman continued to sob, looking down at her lap, where both folded hands now grasped the handkerchief, still unused. It wasn't clear whether she understood Debra's stark report. "She says she has stomach pain. They said she tries to sell her baby, but no one will buy it because they think it has AIDS, like the mother. She says the police beat her up when she was selling her baby. She's afraid now if anything happens to the baby, the police will beat her up again. She asked me to find someone to buy the baby."

With Debra as translator, I tried to obtain a medical history, but the woman didn't cooperate, including when asked about her HIV status. I went through the motions of examining her, but except for malnutrition—bony chest and extremities, sagging breasts, sunken face, and hollowed-out abdomen—there was nothing especially remarkable. During all this time, the woman did not look at her baby, still asleep in Debra's arms. The woman's crying had stopped. Debra returned the baby to her mother, who still did not look at her. The easy part of the visit—the attempted history and physical examination—was completed, and according to the usual, time-honored medical routine, it was time for the doctor to render a clinical assessment and plan, with indicated evaluations and treatment. A gaggle of children from the Hospice orphanage, laughing and shouting, had congregated outside our window. Debra leaned out and gently shooed them away. A warm summer breeze wafted through the curtains into the room. I stared blankly at the woman, who was staring blankly at the floor. Birds were singing outside, and a red-eyed dove softly cooed from a nearby tree.

There was a story here, I thought to myself, but it was much too sad to relate or to hear. I was still dazed, dumbfounded. I'd seen lots of sad, hopeless cases, but this one really seemed in a league of its own. I had no idea what to do. There were no social services I could turn to for help, no case managers or mental health staff—nothing. Moreover, it was a Friday afternoon, and the city was already in weekend mode. Both doctor and patient were frozen, each as helpless and without hope as the other.

"She told me her milk dried up and she has no food for the baby," Debra volunteered, again without discernible emotion. She methodically smoothed out the wrinkled sheet and pillow on the exam table for the next patient. "But she ate lunch here. This woman does not want her baby. Neighbors said she tried to sell her. I checked the orphanage, but they are full. Maybe on Monday they might not be so full." Maybe: God bless them, the Batswana will never tell you it's hopeless.

I mechanically wrote out the woman's meager history and physical exam on her brand-new medical card. She started to sob again, but the baby remained asleep. I had run out of things to write on the card. I looked up at the woman, staring at her as dumbly as she was staring at the floor, oblivious of her baby lying in her limp left arm. I turned to Debra, my voice almost breaking. "Can we get her a food basket today?" I had run out of things to do. Debra shook her head in the negative.

"The social workers have left for the day. But the cooks can make a food package for her. Come Monday, the social worker can get her a food basket and shoes." The Hospice had a supply of used clothing, mostly from expatriates, but the social workers had the keys, so shoes would also have to wait. More out of ritual than anything else—and to make me feel we were doing something for her—I asked Debra to give the woman twenty tablets of cimetadine, an ulcer medication, which was already six months past its sell-by date.

As I watched Debra ladle out the stale pills into a small plastic envelope and write instructions in Setswana on it, I thought back to my AIDS ward in New York in the early 1990s, when I had felt that even though there were no good treatments, my just "being there" and caring for my AIDS patients would somehow make a difference. Back then, I might reach out and touch the patient's hand, perhaps uttering words of hope, often when there was none. But not with this patient. The gulf was too wide.

The baby started to stir. Debra and I helped the woman to her feet, steadying her tenuous hold on the child. Her sobbing had stopped, and she still grasped my handkerchief. Debra escorted them down the hallway, while I sat back in my chair, distractedly bouncing my rubber reflex hammer on the table. The red-eyed dove resumed its pensive cooing. I jumped to my feet, veered down the hallway, and caught up with the three of them.

"Debra, please see if they can help the baby on Monday . . . whatever they can do." My voice was breaking again. Debra smiled and nodded her understanding. "We will collect her on Monday."

I later learned that on Monday they couldn't find the woman in Old Naledi. Neighbors said she had gone off with some men. But the ten-year-old cousin had the baby, who that same day was taken to the orphanage.

―――――

As I later learned, Holy Cross Hospice had once been a retirement home for Anglican nuns. Before that, it had been just another small three-bedroom dwelling in a nondescript residential suburb of Gaborone, which over the years had gradually become dilapidated and run-down. By the early 1990s, the last of the nuns had died, and in 1994 the Anglican Church converted the property to Holy Cross Hospice, named after Holy Cross Cathedral, seat of the Diocese of Botswana. The Hospice relied on an unsteady stream of contributions from outside donors, usually local businesses and individuals, often expatriates. More substantial donors could possibly be attracted, but the Hospice could never afford an accountant to balance its books and verify that the money wouldn't go into someone's pockets. It was not uncommon for paydays to come and pass without any of the staff—the director, two nurses, a social worker, cooks, a driver, and housekeeper—getting paid at all. The Cathedral's Dean, the Hospice's ultimate director, would then cast about and find some money eventually to meet payroll.

The Hospice's neighborhood was much like the impoverished hamlets I saw many years ago in West Virginia. Starving dogs, puny chickens, and little children lazed about, sometimes ambling (the dogs) or darting (the chickens and kids) across the rutted dirt streets. The small brick houses had no fences, save for occasional wire mesh, bent and sagging from the years. Whatever stone walls had once been present had long ago crumbled into ruins. But the community was much nicer and less cramped than Old Naledi, the nearby slum and home to many of the Hospice's patients. For one thing, there was indoor plumbing and running water. TV antennas sprouted from most roofs, and electricity and telephone wires crisscrossed over the streets. Most houses had no gardens, grass, or trees—no sanctuary for much-feared snakes—and the yards were mostly dirt, strewn with rubble, rickety chairs, and old sofas. Residents usually sat out in the paltry shade, the women often styling each other's hair or doing laundry in large tubs, while others looked on, fanning themselves. Some would lie out and nap on mats in the shade. The pace in the Hospice's neighborhood was languid, unhurried. Traffic was sparse, and most people walked unperturbed down the middle of the streets.

The Hospice was not much different from the homes surrounding it. A small ground-level house, it had over the years been converted to offices, patient activity rooms, and a small chapel, where the Dean would hold weekly services. Filling most of the small front yard was a two-room prefabricated building—one room had cots for the sickest and weakest patients, and the other was the doctor's consultation room. In the back, the servant's quarters had been enlarged, and another small prefabricated building had been erected to accommodate tiny offices for the volunteer staff, nurses, social workers, and the director. The property was actually enclosed by a credible wall, with a sturdy metal gate. Although its contents weren't very valuable, they were valuable enough for someone to break in and steal.

The Hospice was not a hospice in the usual sense of the word. Rather, it was an adult day-care center, providing meals, minimal medical and social services, and occasional activities for its clients.

But as with all hospices, the patients were always very sick, many too sick to be helped except with morphine and a prayer. From time to time, a priest from the States or Britain would visit for a few months. In the morning, the van would pick up the dozen or so patients from their homes and bring them to the Hospice, where they would spend most of their time watching soap operas on the TV. Their main social activity was lunch, prepared by two cooks in the kitchen. Later in the afternoon they would be taken back home. For patients too weak to come in the van, Hospice staff would make home visits.

The medical consultation room was very small but functional. Jammed into it were a small medicine cabinet, an ancient patient exam table, a tiny sink, a small desk, and rickety chairs for the patient, nurse, and doctor. The glass-fronted medicine cabinet looked very old, and contained the few available medications the Hospice had to dispense—antibiotics, pain medicines, multiple vitamins, and salves and ointments, most of them outdated, since local pharmacies would often donate their expired drugs. Many of the supplies were donated by various embassies and businesses in Gaborone.

The founder of the Hospice—the person who kept it running for many years—was Dr. Howard Moffat, who also provided much of the medical care there as well. Kind and soft-spoken, Howard hailed from a long line of medical missionaries who had emigrated to Africa generations previously. As superintendent of Marina Hospital, Howard would often work there late into the night, walking the hospital's corridors, trying to find out-of-stock medicines, or treating patients neglected by the doctors and nurses, or addressing any one of the myriad deficiencies of the place. Howard was also a priest at Holy Cross Cathedral, as well as personal physician to President Mogae. Despite innumerable disappointments and setbacks, Howard never wavered in his devotion to the Hospice.

A few months after my arrival, Howard and I met at one of the meetings at the ministry, and we took an instant liking to each other. Soon thereafter he asked me to help him see patients at the Hospice. The job wasn't onerous: for a few hours a week at most, I would stop by and see whatever patients the nurses thought should be seen, and from time to time I'd go with them on their home visits. Most of the patients had AIDS, but there were also uninfected patients with a variety of cancers, usually in advanced stages. And the Hospice salvaged more than a few of them, or else eased their transition into eternity.

———

At the Hospice, it was sometimes easy to forget, as doctors often do, that every patient was unique and special, especially when so many patients seemed so similar. Joyce M. was such a patient. End-stage AIDS, profoundly wasted, alone in a small single-room hovel in Old Naledi. When I first laid eyes on her on a home visit, I could have sworn I'd seen dozens exactly like her before.

"Why are we bothering," I thought to myself as we entered her shack at the outskirts of Old Naledi, directly across the road from a petrochemical plant. With me was Puso, one of the Hospice nurses. Sometimes I was amazed—and concerned—that I wasn't depressed by such forays into the abyss. Was I totally indifferent, hardened to their suffering? Or was my calm reaction to repeated scenes of privation and anguish really a cop-out, a facade? Whether false bravura or a manifestation of inner peace, I should have known, but all I wanted to do that day was see her and move on. I needed to get to gym before it became too late.

On our drive to Old Naledi, Puso said that ever since Joyce was diagnosed with HIV two years previously, she had frequently "defaulted"—missed, stopped, or ignored her HIV treatment and visits to the clinic. No reasons were given, and trying to discern them at this point in her disease would have been pointless. Maybe she had side effects, maybe she had more pressing personal problems, maybe she was depressed, maybe the clinic doctors and nurses failed to impress on her the importance of taking her ARVs, or perhaps she found it difficult to hide her medications—and her HIV status—from a former partner or family members and stopped taking them. Yet for whatever reason, a few months previously Joyce "un-defaulted," and returned to the HIV clinic, which restarted her ARVs. Again, it was a story I'd heard many times before.

Her home was a replay of so many others I'd visited. A massive bed, covered with large pillows and heavy blankets, took up at least three-quarters of the room. Off to the side of the bed was a small counter, on which a compact gas-fueled hotplate rested, along with some plates, utensils, and a few canned goods. A small sink stood in a corner, piled high with dirty dishes. The only decoration was a framed photo at the end of the counter, leaning up against the wall. It was a graduation photo, of a young man in cap and gown. He was smiling the smile of every graduate who is happy his studies are over and that a life of joy and wonder lies ahead. There were many small colleges in Botswana, and the cap-and-gown shops did a brisk business with all the graduation ceremonies. The house was hot and dark, and it took a few seconds for my eyes to adjust from the brilliant sunshine outside. At first, I thought we'd been stood up: I couldn't see anyone there—there was a pile of blankets on the bed, but no Joyce.

"She's on the floor," Puso helpfully pointed out.

Sure enough, there she lay, on a small mattress on the floor, in the narrow space between the bed and the wall. An odd place to be, I thought, and not good for my aching back. Joyce was under several large blankets, and because it was even darker down there and she was very black, the whites of her eyes stood out in stark contrast. I squatted down into the shadows and introduced myself, asking if she understood English, which she did. Without uncovering her, I could see from her sunken eyeballs and gaunt face that she had advanced AIDS. I asked how she was feeling.

"Fine."

*Lord in Heaven*: how many times had I heard the same mono-syllabic reply from similarly desperate patients with similarly dire conditions? In the hospital, patients who were gasping for breath from pneumonia or stroked out and paralyzed from meningitis would, through the fog of their illness, say they were "fine." And when they didn't speak English, the translation from Setswana was the same: "fine." It baffled me, but then again, I was looking at it from the privileged perch of good health. Was it denial, grasp-ing for hope that the bleak circumstances certainly didn't justify? Could it be a calm and final acceptance of the inevitability of death? Maybe saying you're fine would make it so. The joke might be that when I'm on my deathbed, I, too, will say I'm fine. Maybe then I'll know what so many of my very sick patients in Botswana had meant.

So Joyce was fine. But I stuck to my usual routine and asked about shortness of breath, pain anywhere, diarrhea, and so on, more to make me feel I was being professional and trying to provide good care when, of course, no amount of good care was likely to stop Joyce's downward slide. But she persisted in her "fineness," denying whatever symptoms I suggested. She was fine.

Maybe, I thought to myself, the advanced HIV infection had destroyed her mind to the point that she didn't know how she felt. Perhaps she had lost it. It was a fear I myself often had as I journeyed beyond my mid-sixties.

"Joyce, please don't be offended, but I'm going to ask you some simple questions." To see if you're on planet Earth, or perhaps the continent of Africa, or maybe even the country of Botswana.

"Yes, doctor."

"Can you tell me the month and year?" Sometimes I myself had to think twice about the exact date of the month, so I figured I should give Joyce the same leeway and not ask for the date.

"December 2003. I think it's the eighth."

"That's right. And could you tell me where you are right now? Where is this place?" I'd accept either Botswana or Gaborone. "Plot 3545, Gaborone." Geez, I didn't know the plot number, but just getting the city right counted as a correct answer.

"One last question: who is the Vice-President of Botswana?" She grinned.

"Oh, him! The boy! The Honorable, Lieutenant General Seretse Khama Ian Khama!" Like those of ancient Roman emperors, Ian's formal name was long and dynastic. As the son of the country's founding President, Ian was often referred to as "the boy," sometimes affectionately, more lately derisively. And you wouldn't want him to hear you refer to him that way. Ian was very formal, as befitted royalty, the august Paramount Chief of the Bamangwato tribe, the largest in the county.

Joyce had clearly shown that her mind wasn't as ravaged as I had feared, and perhaps she really did feel "fine." I sensed that I probably could have discussed national politics with her—her knowing Ian's full name suggested she might have an interesting past—but I stayed on track. I gingerly pulled back the layers of blankets to examine her. How many times, I thought to myself, have I groped for new words to describe fully what was now before me? "Wasted," "emaciated," "cachexic," "profoundly malnourished"—they never seemed to convey the sadness, the horror, the impending doom. Joyce was almost gone: bony shoulders, prominent ribs, flat stomach, shriveled-up breasts, atrophic pelvis, and arms and legs without discernible muscles. It was difficult examining her heart and lungs—the diaphragm of the stethoscope has to be flat against the patient's body, and the deep furrows between her ribs left no space to listen properly to her heart and lungs, as if it really mattered anyway. Her skin was thick and leathery, almost mummified. I went through the motions, oblivious of her extreme condition. As I mechanically examined her, I started thinking about what might be wrong with her, whether some last-second intervention might spare her. Sure, most likely it was end-stage AIDS, but my job was to "think outside the box," to be sure there wasn't something else going on here, especially something that we might be able to treat.

For Joyce, there were only three possibilities: AIDS, TB, or cancer; or any two, or all three. Her HIV infection was supposedly being treated, assuming she was taking her ARVs and hadn't developed resistance from her past history of starting and stopping and restarting them. She didn't seem to have symptoms of lung TB, but the spread of TB throughout her body was always possible. As for cancer, who knew? The only way to rule that out would be to get some tests, simple ones like a chest X-ray and ultrasounds, as well as doing a pelvic exam and Pap smear. But undergoing these as an outpatient—in her condition—was impossible. And I knew that putting her in Marina—in her condition—was a virtual death sentence, since it would take forever to get any tests done, and Joyce had precious little time left. I stood up and quietly sighed.

Just then, the blankets and pillows on the large bed started to move slowly, as if they had a life of their own. Puso noticed my surprise.

"It is her son. He was taking ARVs, but he had to stop them. The clinic said he has hepatitis. He is very sick. We are taking him to the clinic tomorrow." I glanced at the graduation photo on the counter. The stirring stopped, no one emerging from under the covers. I squatted back down next to my patient.

"Joyce, I'm very worried about your condition. I really need to know: have you really been taking your ARVs or not?" I always liked to think I could make patients feel safe enough to confess to any non-adherence. "I won't get upset with you, but I really need to know."

"I have been taking them, doctor."

"Joyce, I think we need to get a viral load on you, a blood test, to see if your ARVs are working. If they're not working, then we need to change your ARVs. It's the only hope we have." It was possible that her HIV had become resistant to her current ARVs, and that changing her regimen might reverse her course. It was a "Hail Mary pass," but worth a chance.

"Puso will take you to the clinic tomorrow with your son. They can draw your blood test." I accepted her silence as acquiescence. I wrote a brief note in her patient cards, ending it with a plea printed in capital letters:

"PLEASE DRAW A VIRAL LOAD ON THIS PATIENT. PLEASE CALL ME IF THERE ARE ANY QUESTIONS. THANKS!" I wrote my cellphone number clearly. It was my typical, platinum-engraved invitation to the HIV clinic staff to do their jobs.

"And I'll look forward to seeing you again next week!" My cheerful optimism elicited a smile from Joyce.

The next afternoon, Puso called to report that Joyce had refused to go to the clinic. "She said she was too tired to come." I really had no reaction to the news—many patients here, despite their dire condition, refused to follow medical advice or take their medications. I briefly thought about drawing the blood myself, but desisted. I realized that Joyce probably knew what she was doing. One of the lessons I had learned from bungling Comfort's care a year earlier was that being overly attentive was usually lethal. I thanked Puso and said I'd see her the following week.

On the drive to Joyce's house the next week, Puso told me that her son had died over the weekend in Marina Hospital. At the clinic visit the week before, the doctor felt he required admission. "Does she know?" I asked. Often when patients died in Marina, the family wasn't informed. Puso said he didn't know. "Does she have any other family?" I asked.

"Only the son," Puso replied.

Joyce looked weaker, but she smiled and seemed to recognize me. Even though the bed was now empty, she was still on the floor. She was clutching to her chest the framed graduation photo of her son. I dispensed with taking a history or examining her.

"I'm very sorry about your son, Joyce." I took a chance that she knew.

"He is with God, doctor."

"Joyce, we really need to get that blood test. It's very important."

"Doctor, I am fine. I will soon be with my son. I am fine. Thank you, doctor. God is good." She closed her eyes, and fell back to sleep.

Then I finally knew what she meant. Joyce was indeed fine.

———

Some Hospice patients were fun to see. They might be slowly dying from terrible diseases, but they brought a smile whenever I saw them. And I didn't feel guilty enjoying their visits. Such was Ralph, a familiar and happy face during my first months there.

I always knew when Ralph was the next patient to be seen—his approach was heralded by the enthusiastic tap of his cane on the outside pavement, in syncopated rhythm with the squeaking of his leg brace. Although thirty-four years old and malnourished, his AIDS and cancer had paradoxically made him look much younger, more like an adolescent boy. And he had an adolescent's playful temperament. I wondered whether he had had the same light-hearted personality when he was a grade-school teacher, before illness struck him down. Childhood polio had withered his right leg, which was supported by a very old, rusting brace, assisted by his cane

At every visit, Ralph smiled broadly. He always sported a worn, white tennis hat emblazoned with the logo of the Palm Springs Hilton. As soon as he sat down, he'd hand me his medical cards, and would lean intently over the table towards me, as if the two of us were reading them together, conferring about his case as colleagues. However, there really wasn't much to confer about, since for reasons known only to God, he would never take his ARVs, even though he always said he understood he should. Yet despite his rank nonadherence to ARVs, Ralph always kept his regular appointments at

Marina's HIV clinic. He was also a patient at the oncology clinic, where he received chemotherapy injections for his testicular cancer, which had recently spread to his lungs. Most likely, the cancer would do him in before HIV did.

Ralph lived with his older sister, who was on ARVs and who would sometimes accompany him on his visits to the Hospice. A true convert to ARV religion—she had nearly died from cryptococcal meningitis a year earlier—the sister, also a school teacher, had tried her best to convince, browbeat, and threaten her baby brother to take his pills. It was obvious that she loved him very much, and worried about his health.

"This one! This one, he is hopeless," she had exclaimed soon after Ralph started coming to the Hospice, exasperated and disheartened by her brother's obstinacy. "I bring him his medicine, and he always has an excuse—he'll take them later, his stomach hurts, he doesn't feel like it, he's too tired. I tell him how ARVs have saved my life, how he needs to take them to be stronger, and he just smiles and says 'Maybe later.' I tell you, if he was not my only brother, I would . . . I would throw him out!" At the time, Ralph reacted to this tirade as he always did to similar exhortations from me, the Hospice nurse, and the social workers: he would just smile and say that he would take his ARVs. But he never would. Queries as to why he wouldn't were likewise fruitless. It was simply an issue that could not be overcome.

Today, the latest oncology note had bad news: they felt that the cancer was not responding to chemotherapy—the lung nodules were enlarging—and that referral to South Africa for treatment with cancer drugs not available in Botswana was the only option to keep the tumors in check. Presumably, the oncology nurse had started the paperwork for the referral, but there was no note to this effect. This verdict meant that Ralph would die soon from the testicular cancer, and not HIV: such referrals, while theoretically possible, were notorious for red tape and delays, assuming that the Ministry of

Health approved the referral in the first place. I knew that this process would take more time than Ralph probably had left. I thought of Woody Allen's quip that death was a great way to cut down on your expenses or, in this case, the government's expenses. Trying to make such a referral an "urgent" one always seemed to make the wait even longer. Ralph and his family most certainly did not have the money to finance the referral.

Then I had a thought. I dialed Dr. Ndwapi, who was working at Marina's HIV clinic that afternoon. After a brief discussion, a plan was made: Ndwapi would see Ralph first thing on Monday morning in his clinic at Marina. He would then call the Minister of Health, whom he knew personally—everyone in Botswana seemed to know someone in power—to expedite the referral to South Africa. Ndwapi actually knew Ralph, who apparently was also renowned in the Marina clinic for his guileless but obstinate non-adherence.

"Tell him that if he doesn't show up, the nurses know where he lives and they'll come after him with long knives. They've tried to kick his butt before, but he just looks at them and smiles. He drives them nuts," Ndwapi chuckled.

I explained the plan to Ralph and concluded with Ndwapi's admonition not to miss the appointment. "He said he will kick your butt if you don't show up, and so will I!"

"I know Dr. Ndwapi," Ralph enthusiastically reassured me. "He's a nice doctor, like you. I will keep my appointment."

On the way out of the door, Ralph smiled and waved goodbye, as each of us gave the other a thumbs-up. It was our last glimpse of each other. I never did learn what became of him, but his smile and the music of his cane and metal brace will never leave me.

# Chapter 10

# Local Flora and Fauna: "A First-Rate Country for Second-Rate People"

When a friend, a long-time white expatriate himself, described Botswana as "a first-rate country for second-rate people," he wasn't referring to the Batswana, but to his own caste of outsiders who had made the country their home. Botswana's expats spanned the gamut, from truly decent, compassionate people, to chancers and crooks who would steal from their own mothers, to say nothing of looting the pension fund of a defunct company, leaving nothing for its minimum-wage employees.

Initially, in the 1970s and 1980s, the white Africans who had emigrated to Botswana from surrounding nations largely did so out of disgust with the racism of their home countries or to help the country's people. Such emigres included Dr. and Mrs. Howard Moffat, who left Rhodesia because they didn't want their children growing up under the racist regime of Ian Smith. Their daughter eventually did important research in Botswana into preventing mother-to-child transmission of HIV. During the final decades of apartheid, the "good Afrikaners," many of them teachers and doctors, fled South Africa to Botswana in protest against their country's racial oppression.

In addition, many South African students and anti-apartheid activists were exiled to Botswana, again to Botswana's benefit. As a beacon of non-racism in the region, Botswana was the natural refuge for good people, or just halfway honest and decent folk. It wasn't lush or jam-packed with deluxe restaurants, but it was safe and quiet. And, no small thing, it was under the tacit protection of the United States, which was eager to support the fledgling democracy. So eager, in fact, that the Yanks had built an international airport that had a runway capable of accommodating mammoth military transports to ferry Americans out in the event of wars in the surrounding countries. Even today, the good expatriates pitch in and donate blood when the hospital blood banks are bare, especially around the Christmas holidays.

For years after independence in 1966, many of the leading administrators in Botswana's government were white, guiding the young nation in its early years. Although the British left behind minimal infrastructure, they did pass on their legal and governmental institutions. But during their largely benign rule, the Brits didn't engage in much "localization," the buzzword years later for training the Batswana to do it themselves. So at first there were few home-grown people to take control. For example, the first Chief Justice of the High Court was white, an august Queen's Counsel, and his incisive legal rulings are frequently cited even today, but now by Batswana jurists who went to law school, clerked with white judges, and eventually took over. Botswana's first President, Sir Seretse Khama—the country's George Washington—raised eyebrows by openly favoring white expatriates in his government. Since he was black—and of royal blood—he could get away with it without being accused of racism. Even earlier, Sir Seretse had raised more than just eyebrows when he took as his bride a white Englishwoman, an office clerk. He and Ruth Williams had fallen in love when he was staying in London prior to independence. It really was a love story, but the shock back home required many weeks of meetings with village elders before getting their nod. And soon, Lady Ruth's skin color didn't even register with her adopted people.

Over time, the government leadership became less and less white, but many of the once great and mighty lingered in Botswana into their old age. They knew that anywhere in the West they'd be just ordinary people—they would even have to do their own housework and laundry! Once at Caravella, a long-time Portuguese restaurant in the capital, a dinner companion pointed to a table in an out-of-the-way corner. Three elderly white couples, in their seventies and eighties, all very plain and nondescript, were quietly dining. In the States, they could have been retired teachers or plumbers. "Those people once ruled Botswana," my friend observed wryly, but without condescension, since he, too, risked ending up like them, nobodies who once were very important somebodies. "If you stay here long enough, you'll go to seed," he added.

Unfortunately, though, over recent decades Botswana had attracted a much less desirable sort of white people, corrupt businessmen, largely in finance and construction and mostly from South Africa and Britain, with a few from Italy and the Balkans. The boundless wealth of the diamond industry fueled great leaps in the country's standard of living, making Botswana a "middle-income" country, not a basket case like Niger or Cameroon. This money lured many fortune-seekers, some genuine entrepreneurs who added to the nation's wealth and others the type of characters you wouldn't trust with your neighbor's cat, let alone your money. And with the fall of apartheid, many shady Afrikaners—no longer lords of the manor back home—moved to Botswana, where some became feudal chiefs, parlaying other people's money into fortunes for themselves, fortunes which they'd often turn around and lose on some insane scheme, and then remake and then lose again, and so on. Some of their harebrained schemes were beyond belief: a honeybee farm without any queen bees or water, or a road sealant that dissolved with the first heavy rain, or an ostrich abattoir without any ostriches to slaughter, or a cure for AIDS in a so-called mineral dubbed "trizivite," which allegedly was only found on a secret mountain in Namibia but later was used for tombstones *and* cosmetic powder. Some of the braver or dumber expats would dabble in the illegal diamond trade, very risky business that was bound to provoke the local Israeli or Russian mafia, to say nothing of the government, which guards its diamonds the way America guards its nuclear missiles.

The financial shenanigans of these expat chancers always amazed me: they would default on loans, or steal outright—from the banks or their best friends or the pension funds of their workers—and then, after lying low for a while, they'd resurface and do it again, and again. The sort of nonsense that would get them sentenced and imprisoned in the States. I once asked an acquaintance of mine, a rich financier and a character in his own right, why these guys weren't locked up, after being publicly caned.

"My *dear* Dr. Baxter," he replied indulgently over one of the splendid dinners at his lovely home, "Botswana is a *very* forgiving country." Years later, he found out how forgiving Botswana could be, when he was entangled in allegations of financial impropriety. The guy's name was plastered over the newspapers for weeks. But he wasn't publicly caned and locked up, and instead was just fired from his lucrative position at his investment company.

There were also many long-time white expats who, while not shady and shifty, were, to put it plainly, not very nice people—the types who paid their domestic worker the pathetically low minimum wage or, when she fell sick from TB or AIDS, would chuck her out like damaged goods. Through a friend, I knew such a person, an Englishwoman who had come to Botswana decades earlier, initially working at a small hotel and then becoming owner of a brush-clearing company. In her seventies and very ordinary-looking—in England she'd probably work as a clerk—she treated her employees like the rubbish they labored to clear. Whenever a major rain made it impossible to work, she'd dock their pay. Every night after dinner, she and her husband would get drunk, fighting over his ongoing affairs. Whenever challenged over how she treated her employees, she would imperiously retort, "They mistake kindness for stupidity!"

We white expatriates liked to think that we led extremely private lives, our peccadillos and shenanigans kept secret from public glare. But in reality, gossip and innuendo usually left no one unscathed. Unless you were a hermit, talking to no one and rarely appearing in public, you were fair game, and even if you were a recluse, people would make things up—your hermit-like existence would be spun into your being a CIA operative, always a popular rumor, or a sex fiend hosting private orgies in your dungeon, or even worse. Information, misinformation, and innuendo were the currency of the realm among the expatriates in Gaborone, especially during long sessions at the beauty salon, where gay hairdressers would ply gossip between wash, snip, and dry. I will admit that I was as bad as everyone else, wagging my tongue about this or that person, soaking up rumors and scandal, all the while smugly believing I was never the subject of others' wagging tongues. And I will admit to some guilt about hanging out with some of the questionable characters, enjoying their fine meals and witty repertoire—as a droll doctor from New York, I had a cachet that opened doors. But Gaborone was boring and dull, and gossip about Botswana's second-rate people was bizarre and sometimes even true. There was the Marina urologist who claimed to be a foreign spy with his ancient short-wave radio. Or the adult daughter of a prominent businessman who drew great sympathy whenever she related that she had terminal pancreatic cancer, only to be hale and hearty many years later (without treatment), switching her imaginary ailment to an aggressive leukemia. Or Veronica, an elderly American, rich and reclusive, who sold plants out of the back of her beat-up pick-up truck, plants that she had uprooted from public areas in the malls and around the presidential palace. Whenever someone came within a few feet of her, however innocently, she would brandish her right wrist, on which was taped an index card with the written warning, "YOU'RE TOO CLOSE!"

Gaborone was one of the fastest-growing cities in the world, thanks to the diamonds, and many of the numerous construction companies were Chinese. The Chinese were an expatriate community unto itself— most of the manual laborers in these companies were imported from the mainland, living in closed-off, self-imposed ghettos just outside the city, with food imported from the mainland as well. All too often, Chinese construction in Botswana was shoddy—not life-threatening deficiencies, but things like crumbling walkways, parking lots, and ceilings. The problem was that the government had to accept the lowest bid for its projects, and the Chinese were experts at underbidding. But it's one thing to have crumbling walkways and steps, and quite another when the entire country is plunged into darkness, with frequent blackouts—"load-shedding"—all because of shoddy Chinese construction. This disaster happened when the government accepted a Chinese consortium's bid to build an immense coal-burning power plant north of the capital. The plan had been for Botswana to generate torrents of electricity, enough to sell to South Africa and other surrounding countries, which had been suffering major power shortages. But there was one small detail everyone overlooked: the Chinese company had never built a power plant like this before. As soon as it came on line, it blew up, reducing its power capacity to a small fraction of what had been planned. The everyday inconvenience of no electricity was bad enough, but many times Marina's CT scan was down due to lack of power. The newspapers, of course, went berserk, and the government and the Chinese blamed each other for the fiasco. The courts will be hearing this case for decades. The government finally announced it was "bringing in the Germans," a European consultancy that knew about power plants. In Botswana things usually work out, although many years into the future, and the country might yet become the energy powerhouse of sub-Saharan Africa.

# Chapter 11

# All Part of the Package

One of the beauties of life in Botswana was how medical malpractice concerns never crossed my mind whenever someone asked for help—the courts did not look kindly on malpractice lawsuits, or on personal injury suits in general. This was a country where the major cost of auto insurance wasn't the personal injury part—"whiplash" injuries were laughed out of court—but rather was the cost of insuring against car damage from fender-benders and crashes. Unlike the States, where I always had to practice "defensive medicine" to ward off frivolous lawsuits, I was free to do the best I could with each patient I saw. I had lots of time on my hands for clinical activities other than KITSO, Holy Cross Hospice, mentoring doctors in the clinics, and outreach visits upcountry. ACHAP kept me on a loose leash, and any *pro bono* work that was remotely clinical was all part of the package.

Gym Active was my gym, located in an upscale residential area known as the Village, one of the older parts of Gaborone. Perfectly serviceable, Gym Active was one of my refuges, but it was anything but tranquil, always reverberating with deafening pop music. The locker room was usually just as loud—the Batswana bantered and gossiped at the tops of their voices. Although the guys' animated, good-natured discussions were often in Setswana, you didn't have to know the language to sense that most talk was about sports and girls. I largely kept to myself, until one day, a year after my arrival, I had to speak out.

Among the Batswana regulars in the gym was a guy, probably in his mid-twenties, who regularly annoyed me because of his lack of gym etiquette: he never returned weights to the racks, never wiped off workout machines after using them, and always hogged certain stations for what seemed like hours. When I first saw him, he had a beautifully worked-out body, muscular and defined. He usually wore a black T-shirt, on the back of which was printed "No Fear," with skull and crossbones decoration. Aloof and proud, No Fear was always alone and never chatted with others in the gym. Having quickly developed an intense dislike for the guy, I studiously ignored him, always avoiding eye contact during our workouts. He seemed like the type of Batswana—in my experience there were only a very few—who, if ever challenged about his rudeness, would angrily reply, "This is *my* country!"

About a year after I first saw No Fear, I began to notice changes in my gym nemesis: his face seemed to become gradually gaunter, and his arms and legs, while still muscular, appeared less defined. Moreover, his workout pace seemed increasingly awkward, less assured, as he would struggle with heavy weights that many months earlier he had lifted with ease. Of course, it was a story which had played out countless times in New York City gyms over ten years previously, as once worked-out, self-absorbed "muscle Marys" began their gradual descent into oblivion.

Several months after I first noticed No Fear's own descent, as the two of us went about our individual routines, he seemed especially frustrated with his performance. Nonetheless, he pushed on, and settled into the squat machine, right next to a machine I happened to be using. I pretended not to notice how he was panting and strain-ing to push back the 90-pound weight. Just then, his knees buckled in the squat position, and his legs suddenly collapsed to his chest, the weight almost pinning him down. He clumsily steadied him-self with out-stretched arms, barely escaping serious injury. Roll-ing off the machine onto the floor, catching his breath, he looked over at me, and for a brief second we locked eyes, and then just as quickly averted our glances. But each knew what the other was thinking. Before I could say anything, No Fear got up and slowly walked towards the changing room, head bowed, his face etched with foreboding.

I followed my ex-nemesis into the dressing room, and quickly fetched from my locker an ACHAP business card, which listed my cellphone number. No Fear was sitting on a bench, forearms resting on his legs. He was looking down at the floor, eyes glazed. I walked up to him.

"Here! I'm a doctor, this is my number," I barked out in my aloof, no-nonsense "doctor's voice." "Call me if I can help." Further elabo-ration wasn't necessary: I was a white doctor in Botswana at the height of the plague.

No Fear looked up vacantly and took the card. "Thanks." I avoided eye contact, and returned to the gym floor.

At 6:15 the next morning, the sun barely above the horizon, my bedside cellphone blared out Nokia's generic tune, loud and flat. Through my sleep-caked eyes, I tried to see who the caller was, but it was a blocked number.

"Hello, is it Dr. Baxter?" The male voice, Batswana without doubt, did not sound familiar, and, as with most calls from Bat-swana here, he did not introduce himself until I asked who was calling.

"It's Gola." The speaker sounded impatient and annoyed, as if I should know him and what the call was about. "I want to come to you today."

Nothing registered. Was it a sick Hospice patient? Or perhaps a past KITSO attendee, worried about a secret medical condition?

"I'm sorry, but do I know you? Have I seen you before?" The last thing I wanted that day was to see another patient. My morning schedule was full—back-to-back meetings—and I had the Hospice in the afternoon.

"*It's Gola,*" the caller replied, irritated that I didn't recognize him. "You gave me your number yesterday. I want to come to you today." Oh, yes, No Fear. "I knock off at half past four. I can come to you then." Gola was half pleading, half demanding. As with others in the past, the assumption was that I would have to accommodate his schedule. After a minute of bargaining, we struck a compromise: 7:30 a.m.—little more than an hour hence—at the Marina Hospital AIDS clinic. The venue troubled No Fear.

"I don't have AIDS," Gola protested, speaking more to himself than to me. "I need more vitamins to build me up. I don't have AIDS," he persisted. The thought seemed preposterous to him.

"Don't worry about the venue. It's the only office I have. I'll see you in an hour. We'll talk then."

Even before 7:30 in the morning, the parking lot at the Marina AIDS clinic was full, and I had to park out on the street. The clinic was located in a large prefabricated one-story building at the rear of the hospital. Just outside the entrance to the parking lot, vendors had set up shop, their small tables covered with bananas and apples, wrapped hard candy, and cookies. A few tables had air phones hooked up to car batteries, Botswana's version of pay telephones for the poor who couldn't afford cellphones, even if prepaid. Patients had already crammed into the waiting area of the clinic, squeezed onto rows of narrow wooden benches, and a dozen or so were standing outside the entranceway. Many had arrived before dawn, hoping to get to the front of the queue. Others, still clad in heavy overcoats, had started out in the middle of the cold night for the long ride from their home villages.

Inside the clinic's waiting room, a church revival meeting seemed to be under way. Four clinic nurses, attired in white uniforms with pins and shoulder epaulettes denoting their ranks, were leading the throng in a hymn. Everyone was animated and singing in unison—not in wild holy-roller fashion, but with a profound sense of community. After two more songs, the floor was turned over to a local minister, who, Bible in hand, led the patients in prayer, in Setswana, concluding with a scripture reading. Services having ended, the most senior clinic nurse stepped forward and began the daily adherence lecture, delivered rapidly in a mishmash of Setswana and English. It could have been a revival sermon or religious testimonial, except for the interspersed English fragments: "ARVs are not a cure," "treatment for life," and "condomize, condomize, condomize!" The nurse belted out her exhortations like a drill sergeant, the other three nurses looking on approvingly, with their arms folded over their ample bosoms. This twenty-minute session was repeated daily, and many of the patients today had heard it before, on previous visits to the clinic.

I stood near the entrance to the clinic, so No Fear could see me. At 7:45 a.m., no Gola. At 8 a.m., still nothing. I stayed there until a little before 9 a.m., before rushing off to a meeting at the Ministry of Health. I was only slightly annoyed—I'd been stood up a few times before by similar patients. Most likely the venue—an AIDS clinic packed with sick people—had freaked him out.

At lunch, No Fear called back. "I want to see you at half past four." No apology, no explanation for his no-show. Negotiations were resumed, and we agreed on later that afternoon at Holy Cross Hospice, where I was seeing patients. "Absolutely no later than half past four, or I won't be there," I stipulated. I hated not getting to the gym before the crowds arrived and filled up the parking spaces.

Of course, by 5 p.m., well after I had finished with the last Hospice patient, No Fear was nowhere to be found. As I was pulling my car out of the Hospice driveway, a fancy BMW barreled around the corner, blocking my exit. Gola jumped out, extremely agitated. Again, no apology or explanation for being late. Shooting him a semi-perturbed "you've-got-to-be-kidding" look, I motioned for him to follow me to the Hospice consultation room. The medical history was brief: according to No Fear, he was fine, all he needed was some vitamins, and, above all else, he did *not* have AIDS. My exam indicated otherwise—his mouth was coated with thrush, and purple spots dotted his chest and back. Poor No Fear had KS, the AIDS cancer.

"Gola, I'm pretty sure you have HIV"—I didn't use the dreaded "A" word, although the KS made the diagnosis AIDS. "We need to get you HIV tested, so we can start you on treatment." I assumed that his late-model BMW indicated he could easily afford private care and wouldn't have to languish in government clinics.

"I don't have AIDS!" Gola seemed terrified, tears welling up. "My father . . . my father would kill me if I had AIDS . . . I can't get an HIV test . . . " He trailed off and started to cry. I leaned over and touched his shoulder.

"Listen, Gola, what if I got a blood test that measured your immune system? It's not an HIV test, just a measure of your immune system. If it shows your immunity is weak, then we'll get a HIV test, so you can be treated, OK?" Getting a T-cell count was often an end-run around the fearsome HIV test. Doing this in the States without first getting an HIV test was strictly forbidden, a way to lose your medical license. But in Botswana, things were, well, far more relaxed. Circumnavigating the HIV test by getting a T-cell count as a first step often convinced people to take the actual HIV test.

After a bit of to and fro—No Fear wasn't stupid, just transfixed with fear and foreboding—he agreed to my proposal. I drew the blood sample and dropped it off at the lab. I had to assure him several times it wasn't an HIV test. I said I'd call him when it came back in a few days.

"And I will only give you the result in person. I never give results over the phone." Before we parted, I gently smacked him. "Listen, don't stand me up again, and try to be on time. I'm a busy doctor"— I was good-natured—"and we doctors don't like to wait!" For the first time, he smiled. "Yes, I know," he replied sheepishly. "My father's a doctor."

Gola's T-cell count was seventy-eight, abysmally low. When I gave him the result in my office at Marina, he cried, but agreed to the HIV test. Although he had medical insurance, it was through his father's private practice—the clerks there would surely see his visits to a private HIV doctor. So, I arranged for him to be seen in Marina's clinic. He said he wouldn't mind being part of the teeming masses, noting that being just another face in the crowd was probably more anonymous than going to a private clinic.

Over the ensuing months at the gym, we would exchange greetings, but nothing more. And just as I had promised, he gradually returned to good health, bulking up his muscles and hogging the machines and not wiping them off. After a year or so, he disappeared, but I wasn't concerned: Gaborone had a plethora of gyms, and he probably went to one of the more upscale ones. Indeed, the American ambassador at the time created a minor stir by publicly endorsing one of them—pictures of him were included in the gym's promotional ads.

The last time I saw Gola was three years after his brush with death. His picture was in one of the newspapers in a political campaign ad—he was running for parliament for one of the opposition parties. Content that he had already triumphed over a far deadlier foe, I never checked to see if he won.

---

Mercy had been one of the nurses at Marina's AIDS clinic, until she left to work for Debswana, the consortium between Botswana and

De Beers, the international diamond cartel. Debswana had provided ARV therapy for its miners well before the government did, and the care was very good. As with most of us, Debswana's motives were mixed: they wanted to project worthy concern for their employees, but they also needed skilled workers to mine diamonds for Tiffany's and Cartier.

In her late twenties, Mercy had always approached Marina's patients with unflagging warmth, not the haughty condescension some of the nurses showed. But whenever I worked with her, I sensed melancholy, though borne with a deep spirituality. Mercy had been sorry to leave Marina, but pay was so much better at De Beers. Most Batswana nurses were desperate to escape their meagre government salaries, and at the KITSO course and the various clinics they often approached me, asking if I could help them land jobs in the States. I was a potential life raft, a way out. Indeed, the nursing shortage in the West had already lured away nurses from countries like Botswana, worsening the serious staff shortages throughout the country. At one of the AIDS conferences in the States, a researcher—American, white, a "name" in the HIV world, and certainly well paid by his medical center—opined that American clinics and hospitals should stop recruiting staff from Africa, so as not to worsen the shortage of health care workers there. I was livid. In the question-and-answer period, I challenged him for presuming to cut off lifelines for African health care workers. "When you have several children, with school fees and living expenses, making the equivalent of ten thousand dollars a year, then you can tell doctors and nurses they can't come to America to seek a better life for their families." The auditorium, which included attendees from developing countries, erupted into applause.

Early one morning—the Batswana always assumed that if they were up before sunrise, you were, too—Mercy called me. "Dr. Baxter, I need to see you. Can I come to you this morning?" Her voice was freighted with urgency and inconsolable worry, a feeling I had often heard from other patients. I told her to meet me in an hour at Marina.

Mercy was waiting at Marina's AIDS clinic, and we walked to my office in silence. She looked downwards, sad and alone in her thoughts. One of the clinic nurses was at my desk, checking her Facebook page. Flustered and embarrassed, she quickly left. A half-minute elapsed in silence before Mercy spoke up.

"Dr. Baxter, I don't know what to do. I have a great pain in my heart," she whispered, still looking down at the floor with profound anguish. Folding my hands at my chin, as if to pray, I leaned back in my chair and breathed in slowly and deeply, trying to feel the measure of my own soul, to be sure I could bear the sadness I was about to hear.

"Dr. Baxter, I'm pregnant and I can't have the baby." Mercy's voice was breaking slightly, but she continued. "It's nine weeks now. I just can't have it." There was absolute certainty in her tone. "I have two of my own"—she had once told me she had twins, now two years old—"and four months ago my older sister died, and I had to take in her three children. My younger sister lives with me since our mother died. She can help when I'm at work, but she is only fifteen." There was no need to enquire as to what her sister died from. "Two of my sister's children are sick. I am afraid to get them tested, but I know I must, or else I will lose them. My partner will leave me if I have the baby. If he leaves, I don't know who will help me and my children. Do you know anyone who can do an abortion? I don't want to, but I have to."

Abortion, except for extraordinary reasons, was illegal in Botswana, and performing or having one risked jail-time. It was not clear whether referring someone for an abortion, even if it was outside the country, was also an actionable offence. I had always had theoretical objections to abortion, but, regarding it as an intensely personal matter, I had never wanted it outlawed. Nor did I ever try to dissuade patients from having this procedure—never impose your morals on a patient. My only objection was when people here would sanitize it by calling it a "D & C," as privileged white expatriates often did whenever their young unmarried daughters were found to be inconveniently in a family way. Today, Mercy's anguish blotted out any ethical qualms I had. And for Mercy and other women in similar straits, concerns about "when life begins" were just academic, especially when your husband or partner might kick you and your children out of the house.

As in other countries where abortion was criminalized, too many Batswana like Mercy sought help from back-alley abortionists and traditional healers. The gynecology ward at Marina always had some poor woman who had been harmed from a botched abortion. And the medical wards often had women with kidney or liver failure from the various concoctions of turpentine or crank-case oil their traditional healers gave them to end their pregnancies.

After unloading her troubles, Mercy fell silent and again looked downwards, seeming to gaze into a dark and deep canyon of grief. In the distance, there arose the morning hymns from patients and staff gathered in the clinic's waiting area.

"Mercy, let me see what I can do. Give me a minute." I stepped outside the office, into the deserted hallway, and called a physician friend of mine, who gave me the names of two doctors in Gaborone and two just over the border, in South Africa. "The ones in Zeerust charge according to how pregnant she is, so she'd best go soon. I can't vouch for the two here. Sometimes they have complications, so if I were her, I'd go to Zeerust, but that will cost at least a thousand rand and here it's maybe nine hundred pula at last count. It's such a problem, what with the government and all. Let me know if I can help further." My friend didn't ask that I keep her name out of it—she knew many secrets about the great and the mighty here, including their mistresses' D & Cs.

I passed the information along to Mercy, who continued to stare at the floor. "Let me know if there's anything I can do. I hope things work out for you." There was nothing else I could do, no instant referrals to social workers, mental health counsellors, and nicely appointed abortion clinics. And 900 pula was probably the monthly food expenses for her family. Mercy nodded her thanks, and softly— deliberately—replied, "Yes, God is good." She quickly left the room, not once looking me in the eye. *God is good? How could she say that God is good, when her life was coming apart?* I jumped up and ran after her as she was just leaving the building. I handed over the 1100 pula I had in my pocket. "Here, you'll need this. If it's more, I want you to tell me—OK?"

"God bless you, Dr. Baxter."

I hated playing the role of the munificent white foreigner, bestowing largesse on the natives, but I didn't see any other alternative. And God certainly wasn't going to do any favors for her. Then again, maybe He just had.

———

Every so often, I'd get involved in a bizarre case quite different from the "routine" day-to-day patients like "No Fear" and Mercy, as unique each and every one of them was. Although none of my clinical work was boring, I relished those few times I could do something totally different, while still helping someone with AIDS.

An acquaintance of mine—we were occasional dinner companions at a mutual friend's home in Gaborone—asked me to help someone he knew in South Africa. He said this someone was gay, "a little wild," and sick. He didn't want anyone to know about his request, ostensibly because the wild gay guy was a high-level operative in one of the political parties in South Africa. But in Gaborone, there was often a hidden subtext. Married with children and strikingly handsome, my dinner companion was a high-profile businessman and, according to the wagging tongues, swung both ways, especially on his frequent business trips to Johannesburg. Intrigued and always game for a chance to get out of town, I agreed.

From my dinner companion's hushed conversation, it seemed there was yet another "good-time girl" who, after years of wild sex with multiple partners and God knows what drugs, was beginning to wilt. The gay scene in South Africa highlighted the major disparities—a yawning abyss—between its poor black citizens with HIV and their largely better-off white counterparts. After years of denial and downright stupidity, the country was ever so slowly ramping up HIV care for the poor, whereas for many years most whites had had private insurance for their HIV treatments. As opposed to New York City, where the public health authorities had long ago closed the bathhouses and sex clubs, such places flourished in Johannesburg, Pretoria, and Cape Town. Affluent gay men could cavort on the high trapeze of skin-to-skin sex, confident that the safety net of ARVs would cushion any fall. Yes, much had changed since the 1980s.

The next weekend, my dinner companion and I set out for Johannesburg. It had to be by car, because transporting unregistered blood specimens would violate customs laws—better to deal with agents at the dusty immigration offices at the border than at the airport. The lab director at one of the private hospitals gave me tubes, needles, and a cold pack to bring back blood specimens. The equipment was buried deep inside my suitcase.

The immigration office on the Botswana side of the border at Ramotswe, a small down-trodden village a few miles from Gaborone, probably hadn't changed for several generations. An ancient faded sign heralded "Immigration Formalities," which were actually very relaxed informalities. The three ladies sitting behind the desk in the small single-room building, smiling as usual, recognized me from my prior trips across the border. On the wall was a picture of His Excellency, as well as a government calendar and a couple of dated AIDS-awareness posters. No computer to check whether we were terrorists or smugglers. We dutifully filled out the tiny immigration form, they checked our residency papers, our passports were loudly stamped, and out we went.

A mile on down the road was the South African border post. It was more modern, with computers and border patrol guards, who sometimes liked to inspect the trunk of your car, hoping to find contraband they could confiscate, or demand a bribe for. Whereas you could be relaxed and informal with the staff at the Botswana station, on the South African side you were always polite and formal. Whenever you entered South Africa, you felt the difference—you were a privileged white person in a predominantly black country that had endured terrible oppression from white people not so many years ago.

We whizzed through South African immigration and were on the open road, out in the middle of nowhere, into Africa's immense time and space, bounded only by a horizon supporting the blue infinitude of the sky. No billboards, petrol stations, or fast-food joints—nothing except a starkly beautiful landscape of rolling hills and isolated villages, all of which had large cemeteries. As on my past road trips with other friends, there were only a handful of cars and trucks on the road. When we came upon a car on the side of the road, hood up and ostensibly disabled, we didn't stop for the driver and two passengers trying to flag down a Good Samaritan. There were too many horror stories of car hijackings on these lonely roads. This was South Africa: in Botswana, the worst that would happen to you was being robbed, but here you could be robbed *and* killed.

Every so often, we'd pass through a small town—Zeerust, Koster, all with Afrikaans names—which had dicey bars, shabby stores, fast-food squat-and-gobbles, and petrol stations. They all were run-down and sad, like hamlets in West Virginia in the 1950s. Under apartheid, blacks had been compelled to enter stores from the rear and had to be out of town, back in their outlying township, by sunset. Most places also used to have a separate suburb for "coloreds" and Indians, who had higher social status than blacks. Nowadays the towns were mostly black African, with a smattering of Afrikaners, usually farmers.

A couple of hours into the drive, surrounded by bleak, hilly terrain, was a vast squatters' camp off to the side of the road, probably of several thousand people, with tightly packed, ramshackle hovels, innumerable outhouses, and even a community center. More than ten years after the end of apartheid, such settlements were an indictment of the rank corruption in South Africa—the litany of criminality by the highest government officials recounted daily in the national newspapers was breathtaking, but most people just tuned it out.

About three hours into the drive—it usually took a little over four hours to get into Johannesburg—the landscape gradually changed: rural floral shops with charming shaded tea gardens, bed and breakfasts, fruit stands, car dealerships, shops you'd actually like to visit, four-lane roads, and finally upscale shopping malls catering to the middle and upper-middle classes. The suburban sprawl of Africa's greatest city contrasted starkly with the bleakness of the squatters' settlement from a few hours earlier. Carpeting the gently rolling hills of the city's outskirts, stretching to the distant horizon, were immense housing developments and apartment complexes, all boasting affluence, and all enclosed by high walls with electric alarms and barbed wire. As one comfortable largely white community after another passed by, you would think that South Africa had finally conquered its past, that prosperity was everywhere.

We stayed at a hotel in Sandton, one of the city's fancier suburbs. That evening, over dinner, we met Joe, mid-twenties, well spoken, and apprehensive. He looked like a little wet starving kitten coming in from a cold drenching rain, not at all like a slutty sex addict. We had earlier agreed that we wouldn't talk about his medical condition unless he raised it, which he didn't. My Gaborone dinner companion also didn't say much—adept at filling awkward pauses, I prattled on with stories about life in Botswana. But it was apparent that the two of them were good friends, possibly more.

The next morning, as planned, Joe came to my suite, where I had already refashioned one of the long side-tables into a makeshift exam table, covered with blankets. I first told Joe that as a doctor I would maintain absolute confidentiality about his medical condition, not even telling his Botswana friend what went on. A bit taken aback, he said he wanted his friend to know "everything." Then I simply did my doctor's routine, taking a detailed history, including a sexual history, which was as wild as I had expected, and then performing a complete physical exam. Joe's case was an easy one.

"Joe, I think you have HIV. You have thrush"—I motioned to my mouth—"and the rash on your arms looks like a fungal rash which can occur with HIV." Except for weight loss and fatigue, Joe didn't have worrisome symptoms of any life-threatening AIDS condition. I went on to reassure him that ARVs could restore his health in a matter of months. A bit chastened, Joe took the news well. "I guess I should have known . . . I just didn't think it would happen to me . . . I mean, many of my boyfriends and fuck-buddies are positive, but I just didn't think I'd get it . . . "

I suppose I could have thought to myself, *Well then, Joe, what on earth were you thinking when you had unprotected sex with countless guys for hours on end?* But I had long ago accepted that all of us, even though we "know" disease and death are inevitable, think it won't happen to us. At the KITSO course there was a case discussion about a patient who needed ARVs but repeatedly refused, and the attendees would usually say the patient was "in denial" about his condition. I would try to get them to realize that we're all "in denial" when it comes to death. "I know that all of you are going to die someday, but deep down I feel I'll be the exception and God will usher me up into heaven in a flaming chariot, like Elijah." So Joe, like all of us, had been "in denial."

I drew four tubes of blood for the HIV test, T-cell count, and baseline blood count and chemistries. The previous night I had put the cold packs in the suite's refrigerator for packing the blood samples in my Styrofoam carrying container. I also gave Joe a bottle of cotrimoxazole, the sulfa drug always given to patients with low T-cell counts, to ward off PCP, the AIDS pneumonia. Joe's thrush denoted severe immune suppression, and I didn't want to take any chances, even though we'd be seeing each other in a week, when the blood work came back.

Right after an early lunch, we departed for Botswana, so as not to be on the road after sunset. My dinner companion gave Joe a long goodbye hug. Late that afternoon, at the border, the guards could not have been bothered to look into the trunk, and we were waved through. "I wonder how many laws we broke just now," I joked when we were safely within Botswana. Three days later the results were as expected: positive and T-cells of 178.

The next weekend, because we had no contraband of human specimens, we flew to Johannesburg and hooked up with Joe at an airport hotel. I brought along a three months' supply of ARVs, which my dinner companion had bought at one of the private pharmacies—the usual explanation you'd give was that they were for your maid because the government clinics had another shortage. Joe was very calm as I gave him the results. I went over how to take the ARVs and reviewed the side effects. The problem of medical follow-up in South Africa had already been sorted out. I had contacted one of the HIV experts at Wits University in Johannesburg, who would see Joe in follow-up, and my dinner companion had arranged to pay all of the expenses, so Joe's boss, a prominent politician, wouldn't find out from the insurance bills that he would otherwise have had to submit. Flying back to Gaborone, I asked my dinner companion why he had asked me to help, since there were so many other HIV specialists around. "Because I knew you would understand our situation."

At subsequent dinner parties at our mutual friend's home, I would nonchalantly ask my dinner companion, "How are things in Joburg?," and his reply was always positive. It was our little secret. I didn't ask if Joe had mended his ways, although I doubted it: once a good-time girl, always a good-time girl.

———

Some of my extracurricular activities didn't involve direct patient care—"one life at a time"—and instead dealt with the grand scheme of things in the National Programme, although early on, to be brutally honest, it sometimes wasn't very grand.

Four months into my stay, Dr. Ndwapi suggested I attend the ARV team meetings at the ministry. "They need to get off their asses and roll out treatment to other clinics. Marina's on melt-down, we can't keep up. Maybe you can help." Since I regarded him as one of my *de facto* bosses, I gladly complied.

Only a few months after its opening, the HIV clinic at Marina Hospital already had a six-month waiting list of sick patients urgently needing ARV therapy. Without treatment, most of these patients didn't have six months. Already, the fastest-growing businesses in Botswana were the funeral parlors, some of which peddled costly, uneconomical funeral insurance to the fearful. Before AIDS, funeral services were reserved for weekends, but by the time I arrived, they were held daily, the slowly moving hearses clogging up traffic even more. With Marina besieged by all the patients clamoring there every day—many from distant villages—the only solution was to open up more HIV clinics throughout the country. You would think that a sense of urgency would crackle through the various governmental meetings I attended to work on ARV rollout. After a few ARV team meetings, I soon learned otherwise.

Six months after Ndwapi had asked me to sit in on them, I attended my third ARV team meeting at the Ministry of Health. The ministry's modest three-story edifice had been built thirty years earlier, in the much sleepier pre-AIDS era, and a new and much larger building was still several years away. By luck, one of the two elevators in the lobby was working. Taped onto the elevator doors was an announcement: "All staff are welcome to attend a prayer and Bible sharing group daily from 7:15–7:30 a.m. in room 3C."

The small conference room was empty, even though I was ten minutes late. Large cushioned armchairs with heavy wooden frames were crammed around the long conference table, leaving barely enough room for navigation. The mauve venetian blinds on the windows were torn and frayed, the drawing cords long ago ripped out of their moorings. On a wall was the official, albeit ten-year-old, photograph of President Mogae, youthful and smiling. A wall clock, another government staple, had on its face "Now Is the Time to Stop AIDS." The hands had stopped at 4:15, where it had been the two other times I was there. On another wall were several colorful AIDS posters, common fare for government clinics and hospitals. One showed an attractive, smiling Motswana woman surrounded by beaming friends, who looked on approvingly as she was taking her ARVs. The caption announced: "I take my ARVs 100% of the time, do you?" Also taped onto the walls were several Government of Botswana calendars, all from previous years.

The ARV team was supposed to meet to push the national Treatment Programme out to the country's clinics. The "team" consisted of about a dozen ministry staff from various disciplines, including data managers, nurses, and site coordinators. The latter were responsible for assessing which clinics were ready to begin treating patients. The rollout had been plagued by shortages of clinical staff, as well as pharmacy problems.

I found an armchair that was neither stained nor too rickety, and settled in for the meeting. By now a few people had straggled in. An ancient air conditioner quietly droned in one of the windows, barely cooling the room and seeming to have no effect on the overall closeness and humidity of the cramped quarters.

By twenty-five minutes past the designated meeting time, most of the dozen-or-so team members had assembled, including the team chairman, Dr. Ndaba, a retired podiatrist who had also been a newscaster on Botswana TV. The meeting agenda began with a prayer, this time recited in English by one of the nurses: "Heavenly Father, bless us as we work together to help our brothers and sisters who are afflicted with AIDS. Guide us in our deliberations, and let your will be done. Amen." A chorus of mumbled amens followed.

After "Introductions"—most attendees spoke in barely audible tones, making it impossible for most of the others to hear them—came the reports from the site coordinators, most of whom recounted a host of reasons why clinics could not yet begin ARV treatment, in spite of the fact that the ministry had designated them for rollout many months earlier. Each clinic had hundreds of patients waiting to begin treatment, but since the last meeting a month ago, only one new site had begun treating patients. Staff shortages and infrastructure deficiencies remained the most frequent reasons cited, with pharmacy issues appearing to be the most insoluble.

Shortages of doctors and nurses had bedeviled Botswana for decades, but basic health care had always been provided one way or another. With enough resolve and pressure, ARV rollout could move forward, even though a clinic might lack a full complement of doctors and nurses. Another obstacle had been the government policy permitting only licensed pharmacists to dispense ARVs: many clinics designated for rollout did not have pharmacists assigned to them. A proposed solution—using pharmacy technicians in place of pharmacists—had generated heated debate at several of the past meetings. There were many more pharmacy technicians than pharmacists in the country, and they performed exactly the same duties as the pharmacists.

At today's meeting, I asked whether it would be possible for the ARV team to request a waiver from the minister, to allow pharmacy technicians to dole out ARVs to patients in the outlying clinics. Several other members of the team nodded their heads in agreement. "As you know," I added, always deferentially, "pharmacy technicians also attend KITSO, and should be expected to complete it successfully before being allowed to dispense ARVs. Besides"—my tone remained smooth and neutral—"when it comes to non-ARV drugs like antibiotics, there are many clinics where there's only a pharmacy technician or even a nurse dispensing drugs, so it wouldn't be precedent-breaking if the minister were to decide . . . "

"Dr. Baxter," Dr. Ndaba interrupted, beginning to show impatience, "the new minister has been apprised, and we must wait for her to reply. It's out of our hands, and the minister is considering many other issues." Two months ago there had been a reshuffling of the cabinet—the ruling party's politics required it—and the Ministers of Health and Agriculture had switched positions. The new Minister of Health had brought with her many years of experience in dealing with hoof-and-mouth disease in livestock.

The pharmacy bottleneck in ARV rollout also involved problems with infrastructure. Even if a clinic did have a resident pharmacist, it also had to install a number of security measures in the pharmacy area: steel-reinforced ceilings, window bars, security alarms, steel-plated safes, and bars over the doors. The assumption had been that the ARVs stored in a clinic were more valuable than diamonds, and had to be cocooned in layers of security. Many clinics did not have the money for such additions to their ARV clinics, most of which were trailer-like prefabs. At prior meetings, I had pointed out that to date there had been no thefts, or attempted thefts, of ARVs anywhere in the country, including the private pharmacies, none of which had the draconian security measures required for government ARV clinics. In fact, no one could cite any government policy requiring such measures for pharmacies, private or public. Today it was reported that rollout at six designated ARV sites had been delayed solely because of the difficulty in meeting all of the security measures. Each of these clinics had a waiting list of seven to eight hundred patients already deemed eligible for treatment.

"That's a lot of patients," I noted, "and I think we should do everything possible to *increase* access to treatment, even if it risks theft of the ARVs. And this risk is only theoretical—there's never been a theft thus far." Again there were several nods of agreement around the table. Dr. Ndaba shook his head in dissent, almost with pity for the cluelessness of the American doctor.

"I don't know of any pharmacist who would risk his license under such circumstances." This disastrous specter had always been the unassailable trump card, always raised by pharmacists, whenever this issue was discussed. There had never been a pharmacist who had lost his license in Botswana. Knowing it was useless, I did not reply. It was *their* AIDS crisis, I reminded myself for what seemed like the thousandth time.

Next on the agenda was "ARV Patient Reporting." The sites already providing treatment were supposed to fax a report every month to the ministry, detailing the number of patients seen, including the number begun on therapy. Silence. Dr. Ndaba fidgeted impatiently, finally calling on the matron from Mochudi, asking her why her clinic had not submitted a report for the past three months. Apparently the fax machine at her clinic was out of order, and there was no money available for repairs. A new one had been ordered six months ago. These excuses were not acceptable to Dr. Ndaba, who started lecturing her about how the government needed data. The matron glared at Dr. Ndaba, her fleshy arms folded defiantly over her ample bosom, daring him to say another cross word to her. She was having none of his scolding. Rule number one: never ever tussle with the nurses here. They ruled supreme in all of the hospitals and clinics. The matrons were demigods to be appeased, flattered, and cajoled. Over thirty years previously, when I told my mother—a registered nurse from the old school—that I was going to medical school, she admonished me, in the reproving way of a mother who knew her headstrong son too well: "Dan, *be nice to the nurses* or they'll talk about you behind your back!" Well, in Botswana, the nurses would do more than just talk about you: they'd get you reassigned to Siberia.

"We must have this data if we are to advise the minister on progress of the rollout," Dr. Ndaba repeated, this time more as a plea than a threat. He needed numbers to present to his superiors. Estimates were not acceptable to the chairman, even though many sites, chafing under the perpetual demands from Gaborone for data, often just made up the numbers. Most sites did not have computers for data entry, or, if they did, the staff had not been trained in their use. The few ARV clinics that did have computers had found the Treatment Programme's IT system confusing. Whereas ARVs had never been stolen from the clinics, computers frequently sprang legs and walked away. Although the clinics always kept an appointment book, which would tally the number of patients seen each day, they usually did not indicate which patients were returning for routine follow-up and which ones were initiating ARV therapy. But the ministry needed numbers for its IT staff to analyze—the ARV team alone had four such staff. The clinics sometimes obliged, but with numbers that often did not reflect reality.

Dr. Ndaba and the site nurse had reached deadlock. She knew he was powerless to resolve the issue. He knew there was nothing he could do to her. The meeting was now in its death throes. Several attendees were openly checking and sending cellphone messages. Some were semi-stretched out, half leaning on the table in the classic "I've-fallen-and-can't-get-up" posture. The IT persons were quietly typing on their laptops. A few helped themselves to more tea and cookies the ministry's "tea ladies" had brought in thirty minutes earlier. Terminal torpor had set in.

It was nearly half past twelve, the start of lunch hour for government employees. Dr. Ndaba looked blankly at the ceiling as the final site coordinator, another nurse, droned on with statistics from the two clinics under her purview. But just when it appeared the nurse had finished her report, she switched topic to a problem she had found on her visits to her clinics. Near-palpable annoyance with not starting their lunch break on time rustled through the conference room.

"Mr. Chairman," the nurse continued earnestly, "there is a problem with how those doctors are treating their infants. Those people are not giving cotrimox to their babies. I tell them, but they don't listen. They give the AZT, but not the cotrimox. It's a problem." National guidelines—indeed, international guidelines—had stipulated that all infants born to HIV-positive mothers must be started on cotrimoxazole, a sulfa antibiotic, at age six weeks, to protect them from potentially deadly infections, especially pneumonia and diarrheal diseases.

"I don't know how the KITSO course could be more emphatic on this issue," I chimed in. "I do everything but jump on the table and do a flamenco dance to drive home the importance of cotrimoxazole prophylaxis for HIV-exposed infants." Exasperated, Dr. Ndaba sought to end the discussion quickly with what he thought was a brilliant solution. "Why don't you put on the wall a notice about this matter? Then they would remember to do it."

"*Mr. Chairman,*" the nurse shot back with impatient desperation, "there already *are* notices on the walls, over their desks, but they don't look at it. They still don't do it! I don't know how to make them do it. At one clinic, a lay counsellor"—an ancillary worker who had no medical training—"is giving them the cotrimox, but she's giving it at three times the right dose. I tell you: it's a big problem." I resisted the urge to say that the lay counsellor's pharmacy license should be suspended.

"So what you are telling us," an older nurse interjected wearily and half-jokingly, "is that the African cannot follow directions even when it's right in front of him." Nervous laughter softly rippled around the table. The two nurses shook their heads in disgust.

Ignoring the nurse's sarcasm, Dr. Ndaba finally adjourned the meeting with a promise to get back to everyone about the date for the next team meeting, and everyone staggered out to lunch.

Although the pace of ARV rollout in the early years of the National Programme seemed at times glacial and maddeningly bureaucratic, a mere mile from the Ministry of Health was a private HIV clinic that crackled with frenetic activity, unencumbered by interminable ARV Team deliberations and ministry rules. Its director, Dr. Diana Dickinson, was a saint in Botswana's struggle against HIV, a one-of-a-kind phenomenon, a class—indeed, a species—of her own.

Although it's not official—back in the 1990s many private doctors probably had patients with AIDS, but most of them didn't know it— Diana was perhaps the first doctor in the country to treat HIV. A white Zimbabwean who had emigrated to Botswana decades ago, Diana headed up a busy private practice, which employed several other doctors plus ancillary staff. Diana's practice was adjacent to the downtown mall, and consisted of several small, one-story houses, which had been joined together and redesigned for patient care. Its amenities were on a par with a typical private practice in America, including an on-site pharmacy. The privations of government clinics were nowhere to be found at Independence Surgery.

Except for the ones at the private hospitals, private medical practices in Botswana were small, mostly mom-and-pop operations located in residential houses that had been tarted up to look like a doctor's office. Diana's place looked, felt, and sounded like a medical clinic—not glitzy and drop-dead modern, but serious and business-like, at least for Botswana. When I first arrived in 2002, I had had my fill of the mercantile nature of medicine in America, but very quickly I learned that Diana Dickinson was not your typical bottom-line, I-can't-see-you-if-you-can't-pay private doctor. Indeed, she was the complete opposite.

Diana's private practice was "business-like" only in the way it provided high-quality care. Day in and day out, she risked her own skin to help patients who couldn't afford their ARVs. She saw some patients for peanuts—or for nothing—and she provided ARVs from her pharmacy at cost, even below cost for the really poor patients. Whenever the government had a shortage of ARVs, usually due to bureaucratic bungling, she would send over supplies, never being reimbursed for them, because the Ministry of Health didn't have any formal mechanism to repay her. The thought of referring patients with overdue bills to a collection agency was alien to her. Diana would have driven her business manager completely crazy, if she had one. Only much later, when the wolf was at the door, did she finally hire one. Not that Diana was independently wealthy—far from it. Her fees were unbelievably low—100 pula, or around 16 dollars, for an initial visit—and she mightily resisted increasing them.

"Dan, some of my patients can barely afford the fifty pula charge for a routine visit. I can't increase my rates." Although I never heard of a time when she couldn't meet payroll for her employees, I'm sure that, as with Holy Cross Hospice, there were some close calls.

Diana's patients spanned the socio-economic spectrum, from poor maids brought in by their employers, to the rich and powerful, including high government officials. Most had some sort of insurance, but the coverage often ran out after reaching a certain amount, at which time Diana accepted whatever they could pay.

The government had always been skeptical of private doctors. Perhaps government officials might not have held Diana at arm's length if she did not have the nasty habit—actually, it was encoded in her genes—of stridently challenging their plodding obtuseness and, at times, incompetence. Look up in the dictionary "speaking truth to power," and there will be Diana's picture. Slight of build, she always wore trousers at work. Open-toed stilettos arched her small feet to a nearly vertical pitch, which was still not high enough to compensate for her diminutive stature. In her mid-fifties when we first met, with greying hair and aquiline nose, she radiated unstoppable energy and passion for her work. For many years, she worked tirelessly to include private doctors in the national Treatment

Programme, finally pushing the government into creating the Public-Private Partnership.

However, even within government circles, Diana's stature as one of the major providers of AIDS care—and, as I quickly learned, a first-class intellect—earned her unqualified respect. Since its inception, Diana had been on the National Guidelines Committee, the advisory group to the Ministry of Health regarding medical standards for the Treatment Programme. And after getting the government to relent and establish the Public-Private Partnership, Diana turned her energies to changing the treatment guidelines to offer ARVs for everyone, regardless of their T-cell count. Finally, after several years of study—consultants worked out the economic cost and benefit for the country—Botswana adopted the treat-all policy. Although the tide of medical opinion worldwide had supported this move—even the normally conservative World Health Organization endorsed it—Diana's unrelenting advocacy probably played a major role as well.

Diana and I got on well together, and from time to time she would ask me to stop by her office to consult on a particularly complicated case. I always knew the patient would be a veritable disaster, usually very gaunt and wasted, someone whose management would confound the world's experts. It wasn't that Diana's care was at fault—rather, such end-stage patients were usually a tribute to how her attentive care had kept them alive for so long. Many of these people had been under her care for eight to ten years into their HIV infection, and because of side effects and poor adherence with taking their ARVs, they would have a highly resistant virus, resulting in terrible opportunistic infections. Rare was the time I'd stop by when there weren't two or three patients on gurneys in the hallways getting intravenous fluids. Whenever I'd arrive, the receptionists would scour about looking for her—she was always in motion, trying to do three or four things simultaneously. Her concern about her patients always palpable, Diana would usually appear flustered and worried, and as she hastily led me by the arm to a nearby examination room, to her next train wreck, she would summarize the patient's history so rapidly that I had to concentrate intensely on her every word. Her handwritten medical records, on small cards, were immaculate, clearly outlining the patient's course. Her care in documentation had made her practice a sought-after prize for several American researchers, who wanted to analyze her treasure trove of treatment data.

Whenever Diana discussed patients with me at her practice, usually in front of them and their family, she would regard them as human beings, not a collection of medical conditions. It was as if she was including the patient in the conversation, while she related their past history, what the patient did or had done for a living, what the patient's hopes and fears were. Much like the nurses in the HIV clinics, Diana knew all sorts of things about her patients, as if they were long-time friends, which, in a way, they were. Rare was the time I could actually give any advice that was significant, since Diana usually had covered all the bases. More than anything, I think I provided reassurance and support. And, of course, rare would be the time I could escape her office after seeing only one patient. Invariably, she would have several other dire cases in other rooms, and off we would go to consider yet another diagnostic dilemma.

Diana Dickinson was a Botswana original, and an unstoppable life force. I have met few doctors in my career who have touched so many people in such wonderful ways.

―――――――

Many phone calls I received were sad and tragic, but a few of them were funny and almost unbelievable. But then again, it was Botswana.

A year or so into my stay, I gave a series of HIV lectures to the medical staff at the Botswana Defense Force (BDF) Air Force Base, a few hours' drive from Gaborone. It was supposedly the "secret air force base," built with help from America, but everybody knew about it. The BDF provided good medical care to its soldiers and their families, as well as to ordinary citizens who lived next door. BDF officers—doctors—regularly attended the KITSO course, and they were all superb, highly professional and very bright. Doctors from the Indian military, on loan to the country, also staffed the BDF clinics. They all had my phone number, and every so often they would call for advice, as happened one day right after the holidays.

"Dr. Baxter, may I ask your opinion about a soldier here, but it's not an HIV case?" The officer was one of my favorites in the BDF, already a colonel and very smart and personable—the type that could someday become a general—but not full of himself. I, of course, readily agreed, since I had been a general internist long before HIV captured my interest.

"We have a soldier here who was injured in a football game. It was his penis, and he's had problems ever since. He's seen the psychiatrist and the urologist at Marina. The urologist wrote that the patient needs 'penile soothing' and must spend time with his girlfriend. Now the patient is saying he has to live off base and we have to pay for his girlfriend to live with him. Dr. Baxter, do we have to do this? The patient says we have to follow the doctor's order for 'penile soothing,' or else he'll go the Vice-President if we don't." Vice-President Ian Khama was a diehard BDF man—in fact, he had been the head of it, and all of his official photographs showed him decked out in military regalia. It was common for everyone to bypass the bureaucracy and appeal to Ian for help, since he was a micromanager at heart.

"You know, I've never heard anything like that before," I replied. "It sounds like rubbish to me!" I was amused and appalled, not at the soldier, but at the urologist who had prescribed "penile soothing." Maybe he had finally gone moggy after so many years of looking at one-eyed snakes in his urology practice. "Your soldier should soothe his penis himself! If he doesn't know how to do that at this point in his life, he doesn't belong in the BDF!" The colonel chuckled. "And let him go to the Vice-President," I continued. "I bet he'd tell your soldier where to get off!" Ian Khama was no fool and had little patience with fools as well, especially when it came to malingering in his BDF.

# Chapter 12

# Enough Is Enough, or Not Outstaying Your Welcome

The problem with most of us expatriates was that we usually stayed longer than we should. Either we outstayed our welcome, regardless of how much good we might be doing, or we went to seed, growing fat from drinking too much. I didn't grow fat or become an alcoholic, but after a little over six years, I started to feel stale, and at the same time the politics of the place started to wear me down. Besides, the idea behind bringing in outsiders like me was eventually to let the Batswana do it themselves—"capacity building" and "localization" were the popular buzzwords.

I always had the habit of speaking my mind, especially to the other expatriates involved in the Treatment Programme who were building their own mini-empires. I also couldn't help myself when it came to puncturing some of the pretensions of the venerable US Centers for Disease Control and Prevention, which had a major presence in Botswana called BOTUSA. BOTUSA and the American embassy were joined at the hip, and both had major input into how millions of PEPFAR dollars were allocated in Botswana. PEPFAR—the President's Emergency Plan for AIDS Relief—will be the reason why President George W. Bush won't be assigned to the low-est circle of hell for his misadventure in Iraq. PEPFAR has saved millions of Africans from AIDS. Of course, with so much money in play, and with so many American medical centers and AIDS-related organizations in Botswana, competition for a place at the trough was fierce, and the leaders of BOTUSA were very popular people, the Americans with the serious money. Early on, I met Marc, one of BOTUSA's power brokers, who always gave me the time of day, if only because I usually had gossip to share. One of our early con-versations, five months after my arrival in the country, encapsulated America's involvement in Botswana and my own inability to refrain from challenging what I saw as absurdity. During a lunch at Equa-torial Coffee, I half seriously asked him why he was in Botswana.

"Our job is to get President Bush re-elected," he replied in jest, but perhaps a bit too candidly. Such an agenda made perfect sense: it was early 2003 and the election was less than two years away. It would take only a few hundred votes in certain black precincts to tilt the race towards the Republicans. If Bush were to highlight his commitment to AIDS in Africa in a speech at a church in Atlanta or South Chicago, it might sway some of the black middle-class voters, especially if he threw in "family values" and how he talked to Jesus daily in the Oval Office.

Marc then went on to boast how BOTUSA was working with the large brewery in Gaborone for HIV testing of its three hun-dred employees. But he had even grander hopes. "And if we can get BTC on board"—Botswana Telecoms was the country's tele-phone provider—"then we can really get our testing numbers up." BOTUSA was keen to increase testing numbers, to justify the mil-lions they were disbursing in Botswana. That day, as usual, I had to be provocative.

"Marc, tell me whether our prevention messages here in Bot-swana, or any place else in the world, have made any significant difference in the rate of HIV infection. Be honest!" I already knew the answer to the question of whether the CDC's strident A-B-C messages—abstinence, be faithful, condomize—had made even the smallest dent in the infection rate in Africa.

"Not so far," Marc replied with a forced smile. "But we keep trying."

I was tempted to note that one definition of insanity was doing the same failing thing over and over again, but I desisted. All the same, I tried to reason with this insanity.

"We always seem to be looking for the silver bullet, the magic 'behavior-change' message that will stab the HIV vampire through the heart"—I tried to sound sympathetic to his situation—"but none of the research on 'behavior change' will ever come up with the magical intervention. Let me propose a new approach." Marc's smile became less artificial, graciously anticipating another Baxter broadside.

"We've tried the 'AIDS kills' tactic, but fear just makes sex sexier, especially for young people. And making people afraid of AIDS just adds to stigma, and your testing numbers will continue to suck. Why not make our prevention messages ones that affirm sex as a life force not to be denied? Why not have an HIV-prevention campaign that extols sex as the life force it is, but every time you do it, be sure to put a 'thingy' on your 'thingy?' Making 'the beast with two backs' should be condoned, as long as you use condoms." Marc was hardly stupid: he knew there was merit in my ravings. But practical politics would not allow it.

"Not a bad idea, but I don't think Congress and the President would buy it. We have enough trouble just promoting condoms as it is. They're big on abstinence, and we have to emphasize that, if we want to preach condoms." Marc had his own masters to placate, and to get re-elected. Republicans in Congress, beholden to religious conservatives, were adamant in their disapproval of promoting condoms over monogamy and abstinence.

So for the first five years of my stay in Botswana, my sniping at BOTUSA and the CDC was akin to attacking an elephant with a peashooter. I guess my major gripe was the way the people in these agencies acted as if they were superior to everyone else. People in government had a love-hate relationship with BOTUSA: they appreciated the money and expertise, but they didn't like the patronizing attitude.

But in 2008, the year before I returned to the States, I apparently crossed the line, at least in the CDC's mind, by questioning a major clinical research study they were about to launch in Botswana. After that episode, I was probably lucky I wasn't kicked out of the country at the demand of the American ambassador.

Yes, in 2008 I managed to piss off the CDC in a major way. But it really wasn't my fault—honest. I was caught in a controversy between the Ministry of Health and the CDC, one that cut to the very essence of safe-sex messages which the government had been vociferously promoting for many years. The dust-up with the CDC was not of my making, although in retrospect it was part of the growing pains of a major intervention that has subsequently revolutionized HIV prevention in the world. Up till then, the only way to prevent HIV was abstinence, condoms, or sexual monogamy with another HIV-negative person. But in 2008, major clinical studies were underway worldwide to investigate whether an HIV-*negative* person could be protected from getting HIV by taking ARVs—one pill a day to keep the HIV away. The drug in question was Truvada, and one of the CDC's studies on Truvada was soon to run in Botswana.

The problem was that Truvada was also slated to become part of the new first-line treatment of HIV in Botswana, part of the three-drug cocktail of ARVs to suppress the virus. The worry was what would happen if the one-pill-a-day didn't work, if the HIV-negative person taking Truvada still became infected with HIV. If the Truvada didn't prevent HIV infection, there was serious concern that the HIV might become resistant to Truvada and the newly infected person's ARV options for HIV treatment might be compromised as a result, especially any regimen that included Truvada, which was about to become first-line treatment in Botswana. Moreover, this person infected on Truvada might pass on his or her resistant HIV to other people, who might also find their treatment options compromised. At the time, no one knew for sure whether this might happen and, if so, how serious a problem it might become. No one knew, not even the CDC.

Another problem was the way BOTUSA was recruiting people for this clinical trial in Botswana. Most of the subjects were supposed to be young adults, and to entice them to enlist, BOTUSA held several circus-like events, with food and musical entertainment. Up to this point, Botswana's government had been pounding into its citizens the ABCs of HIV prevention. You couldn't drive on the roads, listen to the radio, or watch TV without being bombarded by ABC prevention messages. To suggest that people could have sex without adhering to the ABC prevention strategies was heretical. The festive, free-for-all atmosphere of BOTUSA's recruitment gatherings just didn't sit right with many people in government. BOTUSA assumed that because it was BOTUSA, everyone would fall into line and unquestioningly support this clinical trial, which was really the most radical trial thus far in the country. As with other American initiatives in Africa, BOTUSA probably felt that because they were ultimately doing good in Botswana—and its contributions to HIV and TB care in the country were truly impressive—they could bulldoze their way through with this study.

At the time, I was the secretary of the recently convened Guidelines Committee, charged by the Ministry of Health to revise the country's 2005 guidelines. My job was to move the process forward and organize the complex task of overhauling the guidelines. We were planning to make Truvada part of the new first-line ARV regimen, but the BOTUSA study complicated things. The deputy permanent secretary at the ministry was a really good guy named Dr. Mazhani. A pediatrician by trade who a few years later happily left government to practice and teach at the medical school, Mazhani asked the Guidelines Committee to evaluate the proposed BOTUSA trial, which hadn't yet been formally approved, and to report back to the ministry whether the trial might affect the pending revision of the guidelines. There were rumors, albeit unsubstantiated, that President Mogae—not obstructionist or anti-BOTUSA in the least—wanted this study spiked, since it contradicted all of the safe-sex messages promoted by the government for almost ten years.

Along with other committee members, I had questions about the study, specifically about how vigilant BOTUSA would be in detecting any new HIV infections in the participants and in ensuring that there was no resistance to Truvada in those who did become infected. We weren't infectious disease specialists, but we did have considerable knowledge about the science of HIV. In candor, we had no animus against the CDC study, no feeling that we were going to destroy it. We weren't stupid: we knew that the CDC—*the United States government*—had a major investment in this matter, but we also wanted to be sure that every precaution was being taken to protect the Batswana subjects of the study.

We sent BOTUSA our concerns, along with minor suggestions to make the study safer. They reacted the way BOTUSA always did to criticism, as in "How *dare* you question us! We are BOTUSA!" But they, too, weren't stupid and realized they had to play along, especially since the Ministry of Health supported the concerns. So, they brought over from Atlanta several of their experts to meet with the Guidelines Committee and present the facts about the study. After all the meetings and emailing back and forth, BOTUSA actually agreed to amend their study to incorporate some of our suggestions. Nothing major or costly, but some refinements that we believed would further protect the study's subjects and not make our committee look like a rubber stamp.

Because I was the point person in this brouhaha, the CDC's wrath descended on me. I wasn't a team player, a loyal American.

And to complete my damnation, I was blamed for an anonymous leak to The Lancet, the prominent medical journal, outlining the concerns we had about the BOTUSA study. It never occurred to me to do such a thing, and a few years later, after I had left Botswana, I learned that the leaker was another expat member of the Guidelines Committee. At a subsequent AIDS conference, when I ran into the woman who had been head of BOTUSA during this controversy, I tried to explain the source of this leak to her, but she didn't seem interested in my explanation. Most likely, her mind, like that of the CDC, had been made up: I was a troublemaker.

Ultimately the BOTSUA study went forward, and, like several other prevention studies using Truvada, it showed that a pill a day actually did prevent HIV infection, without causing complications or resistance in those few who did become infected on it. Nowadays, pre-exposure prophylaxis—PrEP—is the standard of care, and has saved thousands upon thousands of high-risk people, especially young gay men, from HIV infection. But in 2008 we didn't know this.

When I announced I was leaving Botswana in late December 2008, the Batswana said they were sad to see me go—there were the usual reactions of shock and disappointment, as in "Why are you abandoning us?" But in Botswana, things were multilayered: they, too, knew that it was time for me to go. The two Batswana I respected most, Drs. Gaolathe and Ndwapi, expressed regret, but didn't try to persuade me to stay, since they knew they could get along perfectly well without me. By then, expats like me were akin to trainer wheels on a bicycle when the bicyclist had long ago learned how to ride without them—it was nice to have the trainer wheels, but they really weren't needed any longer.

Besides, after years of fits and starts, after years of stubborn matrons and obstinate pharmacists complaining about not having enough staff or enough security bars on the clinic pharmacies, the National Treatment Programme was afloat, no longer taking on water and lurching aimlessly. Tens of thousands were on treatment, among the blessed fold of the spared, and HIV clinics were opening in the remotest parts of the country. Despite the mind-numbing ARV team meetings that seemed to go nowhere, despite a multitude of apparent impossibilities, the Batswana were finally doing it. The great "experiment"—whether Africans could treat AIDS by themselves—had been settled.

In retrospect, I have often wondered whether Botswana's Treatment Programme should be judged by the many lives saved or by the many lives lost from the delays and turf battles of the early years. Yet when you look at the big picture, when the definitive history of this never-before initiative is finally written many years from now, people will remark how amazing it was that the country didn't implode into chaos and its people didn't go totally mad. Within a few short years, a small, sleepy country—Africa's version of Switzerland—had absorbed two simultaneous blows of epic proportions: AIDS, with all of its fear and suffering, and an invasion of hordes of us people from the West, with our hysteria about getting people on ARVs immediately, without delay. For eons, the Batswana had survived by addressing problems in a deliberative, consultative manner, whereas we Westerners stressed speed and deadlines, and tried to beat the Batswana over the head with our frenzied approach to AIDS. The Batswana had to face two tsunamis at once—AIDS and us crazy people from the West. Perhaps Dr. Ndwapi's sage retort to criticism of Botswana's embracing opt-out HIV testing—"It works for us"— might also be his response to criticisms of the sometimes chaotic and slow way his countrymen initially confronted their AIDS crisis: it worked for them.

On my day of departure, as I walked to the small Air Botswana airplane that would ferry me to Johannesburg for the long trip home, the cumulous clouds seemed especially fluffy and playful, buoyed up by the late afternoon's warm breezes. Their serene, majestic processions had lifted up my spirits so many times over the years. After take-off, I periodically peered back from my window seat towards Gaborone, straining to see it one last time before it disappeared into the murky dusk. During my journey home, a kaleidoscope of past patients streamed through my consciousness . . .

Thapelo—"Prayer"—the promising University of Botswana student, active in campus politics and about to graduate, suffocating to death from AIDS-related pneumonia, whose suffering I wanted to remember when my time came . . .

Matilda, the head nurse of Molepolole's HIV clinic, who had gradually slipped away, never HIV tested, shrouded in her dark blue nursing cloak—red AIDS ribbon prominently attached—that reminded me of my mother's nursing cloak from many years past . . .

Joyce, waiting to die from AIDS in her Old Naledi hovel, clutching her dead son's graduation photo and reassuring me that she was "fine" . . .

Joe, the "good-time girl," whose fall from the high wire of skin-to-skin sex was halted by ARVs . . .

Ralph, the Hospice patient with AIDS and testicular cancer, playfully tapping his cane in rhythm with the creaking of his rusted leg brace as he strode towards the consultation room . . .

The family of five in the Molepolole clinic, held together by the indomitable love and courage of the mother, their rock . . .

And of course, Comfort, who taught me that in Africa it was best to use the light touch, to step back and let things work out on their own . . .

Plus Polite, whom I just should have taken by the hand to be HIV tested when she was pregnant . . .

As I reflected on my legion of patients, I was confident that I had been witness to great suffering, and with this realization was a proud—smug—feeling that the suffering of most American patients was trivial in comparison. It was the seed of my near-destruction three years later. Little did I know that my nearly six-and-a-half years in Botswana were merely a prelude, a preparatory rehearsal for my later two years there, when I would come to a new awareness about myself, my patients, and the suffering that all of us endure.

But first I had to spend four unhappy years in the wilderness of American healthcare. It would be the lowest point of my life.

# PART 3

# AMERICAN INTERLUDE

# Chapter 13

## Room 4224

Three years after I had left Botswana and returned to New York, I was lying in a hospital bed in room 4224 in the neurology unit of the University of Cincinnati Medical Center, bleakly staring at the ceiling and at my own imminent mortality. I was waiting for X-ray results—did I have a malignant brain tumor?—that might well announce my demise. I calmly reflected on my life, and wondered whether I'd ever see Botswana again.

When I was in Botswana, people would sometimes ask if I missed the bright lights of New York, where I had lived since 1992. Oddly enough, I didn't, maybe because I knew I could visit frequently, which I did, and because I knew I'd eventually return there for good. Unlike some of the Americans in Botswana, I never thought of staying in Africa indefinitely. Never one to take even a brief time-out, within a few days of my return to the city I resumed working at the Ryan Center, the community health center in Manhattan where I had previously been medical director, only this time I had the more exalted title of Chief Medical Officer of our entire network, which included four clinics. As before, we cared for the poor, the uninsured, the undocumented immigrants. But I didn't want to lose touch with my former home in Africa.

Right before I left Botswana, I thought I had worked out an arrangement with the Ministry of Health to work, *pro bono*, as a consultant to the Guidelines Committee, to help with any issues arising from the 2008 revision of the guidelines, which I had been a major part of. I had hoped to stay involved with the Treatment Programme by email, phone calls, and occasional visits, at my own expense. A month before my departure, I submitted a "Terms of Reference," outlining my proposed role as a consultant, which I thought had been approved by the ministry. A few weeks after my return, I received a major smack-down email from one of the higher-ups in the ministry's ARV office—along the lines of "Who do you think you are?" I was hurt and stunned, but realized that most likely one of the Americans lingering there had decided there should be only one HIV expert on the committee. I really wasn't surprised.

I did, however, return to Botswana four months later, to head up a final Advanced KITSO course. After I had been in Botswana for a year or so, I concluded that an advanced HIV course was necessary to develop HIV specialists—Batswana doctors who could do what I and other expats were doing. Harvard and ACHAP were both behind it, and we held the Advanced course every few months for those doctors who wanted to become HIV experts. As I would tell the participants, it was the sort of course that could be given in New York City, one that didn't pull punches or dumb down the topics. My return visit went well, until I learned what had happened with Polite, my housekeeper of over six years.

Once Polite and her baby boy started ARVs, they thrived. They were testimony to the curative powers of the new HIV treatments—in fact, Polite was even featured in one of ACHAP's newsletters. Over the years, I continued to supplement her salary, pay for the gas for her stove, and, eventually, pay for Paul's preschool and kindergarten fees and supplies. I felt I owed her—actually, Paul—a bit more than usual. Polite took the news that I was leaving very hard, with lots of tears. Before I left, I set up a savings account for her at one of the banks and deposited five thousand pula in it. A friend of mine gave her a job at his construction company, and his personal assistant, warm and welcoming, accommodated Polite and her family in the servant's quarters at her house, close to her new job. Polite was set up: a job, free housing, and money in the bank, plus free HIV care in government clinics and free public education for Paul.

When I went back to Botswana to do the Advanced KITSO course in early 2009, the full scope of Polite's collapse became apparent. My friend had already emailed me disquieting news. First, Polite quit her job and was working at a factory. More worrisome, on weekends and several week nights, she would spend long hours at her church and leave Paul, only six years old, alone in the servant's quarters, causing her host and the neighbors a lot of worry. And there was only sixty pula left in her bank account. Before returning to New York after the Advanced course, I confronted her with these problems and asked her what had happened to all the money. She just shook her head sadly, saying she didn't know.

My failed attempts to provide for Polite reflected the unsolvable problem of being a "rich" white expat trying to be good to people who were poor and who viewed money and largesse from a different perspective. Polite and I bade each other farewell, knowing that the relationship had finally ended. The fob-off by the Ministry of Health and the situation with Polite had disappointed me: I really didn't want anything more to do with Botswana.

At the Ryan Center, I was once again submerged in the dark world of the American healthcare system. It was more hellish than I had ever expected. The people at Ryan were absolutely wonderful, unfailingly kind and supportive—if it weren't for them, my meltdown would have happened much sooner. The soul-numbing inanities, insanities, and wastefulness of healthcare had only become worse. As I grew older, I found it increasingly difficult to stomach hypocrisy, and the healthcare system was rife—malodorously rank—with hypocrisy. There was an army, akin to an immense swarm of locusts, of consultants, quality improvement experts, administrators, and government bureaucrats. Legions of nurses, who had never touched a patient after nursing school, administered absurdly complicated programs with neo-Orwellian names like "Patient-Centered Medical Home" and "Meaningful Use of Electronic Health Records." In fact, all these programs did was burden health centers like Ryan with countless, redundant tasks that really didn't improve patient care. At meeting after meeting with these people, I had to paste on a smile and pretend to be interested, when deep down I had nothing but contempt for what they represented, for what they were doing to health care.

As opposed to Botswana, where I reveled in patient care, I no longer found solace treating patients during the half-day session I had each week. The only reason I continued as Chief Medical Officer was that I thought I couldn't deal on a daily basis with America's whining patients with their seemingly petty complaints. I'm sorry, Ms. Jones, I know your knees hurt, but they really weren't made to carry 350 pounds of blubber. Mr. Jones, I know you have a tension headache from your job, but if you'd like to experience a real headache, try cryptococcal meningitis from AIDS. Or, I'm sorry your HIV entitlements don't cover weekly acupuncture and aroma therapy—how would you like to get by each month on a paltry food basket of flour, canned goods, and vegetables? Of course, I never said such things, since otherwise they'd run complaining to my boss. I was smug in my belief that in Botswana I had seen *real* suffering and privation, not the largely minor aches and pains of my patients in New York. When I was in Africa, I often flamed off that "I never want to treat another American on American soil," but there I was, back at it, dealing with what I regarded as demanding, entitled patients in a healthcare system that was dysfunctional beyond words and beyond repair.

A little over three years after my return to New York, I was finally struck down by a major paroxysm, precipitated by one job stress too many. At that point in my unhappy sojourn at Ryan, anything could have laid me low—an obnoxious patient, one meeting too many—but it ended up being an ugly argument with my boss, whom I admired and loved. I left her office shaking, terrified that I had finally crossed the line, that I would be sacked. The next day, a Saturday, I was in Ohio with my family, still stressing out big-time over our fight. The last thing I remembered that afternoon was driving into the parking lot of the local gym; the next thing I recalled was waking up several hours later in the emergency room of my hometown's small hospital, my two worried sisters sitting at my bedside. The nurse was giving me another intravenous push of labetalol for my dangerously high blood pressure of 200/120. I felt fine, with excellent memory of everything, except that the prior three hours were a total blank.

The presumed diagnosis was transient global amnesia—TGA for short—where your focus is so constricted that you live literally from moment to moment and cannot recall anything from the past until you snap out of it. Emotional stress and physical exercise—at the gym I had both—are often precipitating causes. Apparently I had driven to one of my sisters, upset and claiming my blood sugar was low. When a gallon of orange juice didn't cure me, they took me to the emergency room. Although my head CT and other tests were negative, they decided to ship me off to the University of Cincinnati's neurology unit for further evaluation.

That night, in rapid succession, I saw the unit's medical student, resident, and fellow, all of them asking me the same questions and doing the same exams on me. The next morning, I had an MRI. An hour later, the neurology specialist, young and very accomplished, stopped by. He reviewed my history, exams, and labs, and said he concurred with the diagnosis of TGA. But then an ominous caveat.

"I looked at your MRI and it seemed fine, but there's an area I want to review with the neuro-radiologist. He just came on duty, and I want to go over it with him. Should take only ten minutes, I'll be right back." I knew it. Up till then, everything had been fine, everything completely normal, but now, at the last minute, there was a glitch, a problem. An aneurysm? An infiltrating glioblastoma, the most dreaded of brain tumors, which kills in a few months after diagnosis? I felt that my previously charmed life was about to come crashing down.

Lying in my bed in room 4224, waiting for my neurologist to return with news that might well mark the beginning of my end, I was actually able to live in the moment—I accepted that there was absolutely nothing I could do to cajole, placate, or nudge the fates to allow me to live beyond my allotted time. During those minutes, I thought about the myriad patients I had cared for at St Clare's and in Botswana, people who faced terrible conditions and eventually died from them. I appreciated the irony of how, after decades of delivering bad news to patients and their families, I could now be on the receiving end. I was no different from my patients, no more special. My reverie was abruptly interrupted by the neurologist, who whisked back into my room.

"MRI's fine. I want to keep you overnight and if you're OK, you can go home tomorrow. Just to be complete, I want them to do a lumbar puncture on you." We briefly discussed my diagnosis— I had already looked it up on the hospital's internet—and he was off. At that moment, I felt such a state of grace. I quietly cried, but my mini-catharsis was interrupted by the entrance of my resident with spinal tap tray and young medical student in tow. Somewhat sheepishly—they knew I was a doctor—they asked if they could do a lumbar puncture and if the student could try first. I may have lots of faults, but having a double standard in such instances was not among them. I promptly rolled over on my side, scrunched my knees to my chest, and pulled back my flimsy hospital gown to get it over with.

"When I was a medical student, the old saying was 'See one, do one, teach one,' but usually it was 'See one, *mess up one*, do one, teach one.'" They pretended to be amused. Well, I was right about messing up: the medical student impaled me three times before the resident took over and quickly extracted crystal-clear spinal fluid. The student was mortified, and I did my best to reassure him. "Don't worry," I joked, "I'm sure the jury will award me several million for pain and suffering."

The next day I was discharged—the spinal fluid was negative—and the following day I was back at work at Ryan. My deeply concerned boss had called me several times during my hospitalization, and we made up as usual. I knew things were fine between us when, despite her telling me to take the week off, I showed up for work and, pretending to be pissed off that I had returned so soon, she dryly greeted me with, "You're an asshole." It was her way of saying she still loved me.

My TGA and brush with my mortality in room 4224 tamped down my over-the-top reactions to the insanity of my job, and convinced me that I had to get out. But where to? I hated medical administration, and I thought I hated direct patient care as well. The only time I had been truly happy in my work was amid the craziness of St Clare's and Botswana, where I could just provide the best care I could, without worrying about mindless regulations and bureaucracy. There were no longer places like St Clare's in the city –thankfully—and I had been sour on Botswana ever since the Ministry of Health had nixed my being a consultant. I thought that my experience in Botswana would easily land me a job somewhere else in sub-Saharan Africa, but after nine months of searching, I found nothing. Most likely, they thought I was too old.

Then, in late 2012, I heard that the University of Botswana had vacancies in its medical school, which had opened a few years earlier and, as was often the case there, was struggling. Sending numerous emails and completing copious forms—and I suspect Dr. Ndwapi, always generous and supportive, put in a good word for me as well—I landed a two-year contract as lecturer in the medical school. Just as when I accepted the job in Botswana in 2002, I had no idea what my new job entailed. But it was away from American healthcare. After a fruitless search for jobs in Africa, Botswana was the only place that would have me. There was probably a joke somewhere in this fact.

Yet when I returned to Botswana in July 2013, I still had smug contempt for American patients, a burden that only a year earlier had propelled me to room 4224. I was certain that the suffering of most American patients was inferior, trivial compared with that of Africans, who had to face their own anguish with little or no support or succor. Little did I know that my next two years in Botswana would finally exorcise my arrogance, extinguishing it in the real belly of the beast, Marina Hospital, where I would care for the sickest, most desperate patients I had ever seen in my life. I emerged two years later a changed person and a changed doctor.

# PART 4

# BOTSWANA, 2013–2015 INTO THE BELLY OF THE BEAST

# Chapter 14

# The More Things Changed . . .

A cardinal rule about writing is to avoid clichés—those lazy, overused phrases lacking originality—but when I returned to Botswana in mid-2013, after an absence of four years, my reaction, however clichéd, was that the more things had changed, the more they remained the same, but in a very Botswana sort of way. Many of the potholed two-lane roads wending through the busiest parts of Gaborone had been replaced with well-paved four-lane roads. But the driving was as crazed as before, possibly worse, since the extra lanes were invitation to speed and weave in and out of traffic, often with disastrous results. In the new central business district, previously a large tract of empty bush, several new buildings had sprouted up, including the Labor Court and two twenty-six story apartment complexes, Botswana's first skyscrapers. But the Labor Court was a ponderous, out-of-proportion monstrosity with faux columns surmounted by odd, disjointed neo-classical pediments— it was a monument to banal Chinese architecture. The apartment buildings were supposed to be deluxe properties, but many of the units were cramped and dark—there were recurrent rumors that one the properties was in trouble. The nearby government compound boasted a new ten-story Ministry of Health, where the elevators were as slow as the old ones, every morning still started with group prayer, and the tiles in the foyer were already coming loose. The pula had continued its downward slide, not a good thing since my salary was in pula. Because of inflation, there were now two hundred pula notes—previously, hundreds were the largest. Ian Khama, now president, addressed the high cost of food by helpfully suggesting that people grow vegetables in their gardens. Of course, the Daisy-Loo saga occasionally popped up in the newspapers— Batswana will be colonizing Mars before that mess is cleaned up. My new driver's license was no longer "good for life," now expiring in five years, and on the application I wasn't asked whether or not I was an imbecile. But reapplying for my medical license at the Health Professions Council took three visits to its dingy out-of-the-way office before its faltering computers finally spit mine out. But thankfully, the Batswana were the same as when I had last lived there: warm and welcoming—and still very much their own people.

As a lecturer in the new medical school, I was at the bottom of the academic pecking order, akin to being a teaching assistant at a university in the States. The medical school, slated to graduate its first class of doctors a year after my arrival, was part of the much larger University of Botswana, the country's premier university, which every year churned out several thousand graduates, including several hundred lawyers, most of whom couldn't find jobs and ended up working as security guards or herding cattle in their home villages. There were also hundreds of degrees in the hospitality industry and social work, again with only a handful of jobs available in the country. However, Botswana did need doctors, since few of the young Batswana the government sent to medical schools outside the country ever returned home to practice, so lucrative were the jobs elsewhere. Drs. Gaolathe and Ndwapi were the most notable exceptions. The new medical school—housed in a gargantuan, gleaming building equipped with the latest technology—was supposed to solve this problem.

When I was in Botswana the first time, there was technically a medical school in the university, at least on paper, and it had a "Founding Dean," a highly regarded American physician. He laid the groundwork for the eventual opening of the school, but he somehow had irritated the university's authorities, who were rumored to have a very dim view of doctors, especially ones who felt they should be paid more than anyone else. The disagreement came to a head when they slashed the Dean's salary—politics in Botswana were never pretty. Disgusted, the Dean left the country, and since then there had been only an Acting Dean, an older Italian, who was also beaten down by his bosses.

Although I did lecture from time to time in the new medical school building, almost all of my teaching was based at Princess Marina, Botswana's big referral hospital, where the third- and fourth-year students were assigned clinical rotations, including the medical wards. At Marina, I attended Morning Report, met with the students and residents for formal lectures and bedside teaching, and—most important—served as "specialist" attending physician on the medical wards, supervising a team of students, interns, and residents caring for desperately sick patients. For the most part, the interns, residents, and, above all, the medical students were bright, motivated, and dedicated to their patients. Besides, they always laughed at my jokes.

Marina sometimes stretched to the limit the students' ability to cope with some pretty sad moments. Part of their ward rotation was weekly "Bedside Teaching," where a student would discuss one their team's patients with me and the other students. Once, a student presented the case of a twenty-eight-year-old man, a security guard, who had been admitted a day earlier for severe pneumonia. Never before HIV tested, he tested positive the night of admission—a common scenario even this late into the National Treatment Programme. In her presentation, the student described purplish KS spots coating the patient's skin. "This is a good case," I thought to myself, because there were many possible causes of his pneumonia—we could thrash out the "differential diagnosis," the list of possible diagnoses. But first we set off to the patient's bedside, so I could go over the patient with the students and point out findings on the physical exam. My student confidently led the way, with me right behind her, with the others, as they often did, trailing in the distance.

As soon as we got to bedside, I knew our discussion would involve more than the differential diagnosis. The poor guy, very wasted and covered head to toe with KS spots, was dead. It happened often at Marina—the nurse or even the family would find the patient dead in bed. Initially looking forward to sharing her patient with us, my student suddenly froze with shock: the man whom she had seen alive earlier that morning on rounds was no more. As the others assembled around the bed, their lighthearted banter abruptly ended. These students were three years out of high school—there was no four-year college before enrolling in the medical school. Most of them were twenty or so, and were just beginning on the Marina wards. My student's face was etched with worry and sadness, but no tears, although I'm sure she wished she could cry. Her colleagues were likewise chastened, taken aback at seeing death, for some of them for the first time. I motioned for them to step back into a quiet corner of the ward.

"Guys," I said softly, "this was someone's son, or brother, or husband, or father. From the looks of him, he probably didn't have a chance anyway. Some people might blame him for not seeking care earlier, not getting HIV tested, but until you're perfect, don't judge patients like this. He probably had a universe of fears. Maybe he had actually tested positive a long time ago, but was too terrified to do anything about it. But I do know this, that during his last day on this earth, he received kindness and caring from your colleague"—I nodded towards my student, who was holding back the tears—"and that's really what medicine is all about, kindness and caring. Yes, you need to know some medicine, and in just a moment we'll discuss the differential diagnosis of his pneumonia. But never forget that every patient is unique and special." I doubt if many college-age students in the States could have stood up to the daily onslaught of suffering and death that my Batswana students endured.

Yes, the more things changed, the more they remained the same. When I started at the medical school, I thought that I'd see only the occasional patient with end-stage AIDS. After all, the HIV/AIDS Treatment Programme had made tremendous strides in getting up to 90 percent of eligible patients on treatment. But I was wrong: legions were still being admitted to hospitals with AIDS. Either they hadn't been HIV tested, or else they had tested positive and, for whatever reason, had fallen through the cracks, never getting treatment. Death had definitely not taken a holiday, not even a brief break.

# Chapter 15

# Princess Marina, I

It was never quite clear when Princess Marina Hospital acquired the reputation of being a place where people went to die from AIDS. But sometime in the first decade of this century, as HIV was engulfing Botswana, Marina was too often a stop on the way to the back of a hearse. Yes, some patients, even very sick ones, did improve and survive, but the monthly mortality rate on the medical wards always hovered around twenty percent. One in five patients never made it out alive.

Built in different phases, Marina was the country's major medical center, a government hospital available to any citizen in need of care. Located in the heart of the capital, it had become a sprawling complex that dwarfed all the other hospitals in the country. Except for the large three-story administration building, the wards and ancillary buildings were single-story, all interconnected by covered walkways. The various specialty wards—medicine, surgery, orthopedics, obstetrics, gynecology—were largely the same: every ward was divided into five large cubicles, each of which was crammed with ten beds, sometimes more when overcrowding required mattresses on the floor and in the main hallway. The male and female medical wards had two smaller rooms for TB cases, with three beds in each. As with any large hospital, there were lab, radiology, operating suites, an ICU, and a busy emergency room, plus a very large morgue.

When I arrived in Botswana in 2002, Marina already looked very worn and dated, and the dark brown and green paint on the wards' walls made the place look even older than it was. Patient beds were very old, with flimsy mattresses, many stained. Bedding consisted of just one sheet; blankets, a necessity in Botswana's chilly winters, were often the patient's responsibility. Frequently there were no patient gowns, and many patients were in their street clothes. Privacy curtains on the wards had largely disappeared, with the few remaining ones ripped and torn. The hospital kitchen did serve three meals a day, but the food was monotonous. At their bedside, many patients stored snack foods, fruit, and juice brought in by their families. There was no air conditioning, only overhead ceiling fans. Bedside stands, chairs, and furniture at the nursing stations were all ancient.

But the place was clean, never squalid, and for the most part it wasn't falling apart, save for the rare ceiling fan that would crash to the floor without warning. Outdoor public areas had shrubbery and nice landscaping, although the signs exhorting "Put Litter in Its Place" had no trash bins nearby. Every Christmas, the wards would be festooned with holiday decorations, which would usually remain in place until February or March. Bathrooms in the three-story administration building always had toilet paper, soap, and paper towels, but the wards' group bathrooms would always run out of these amenities. But despite all this and the drab, 1960s feel to the place, Marina really didn't look like a dump. The infrastructure was there. It had the potential to be a real hospital, even a good hospital.

During my first stint in Botswana, I only had minimal contact with Marina, usually looking in on patients for friends, never actually taking direct responsibility for the medical care. Maybe back then I sensed that I wasn't ready for such raw, heavy-duty challenges in what was often a valley of darkness only briefly pierced by light. But now, as a lecturer, I had no choice. I often would quip that at Marina we doctors were trying to make a car run with three wheels. Or that we were simply going through the motions of providing medical care, albeit in very, very slow motion. The real challenge was not to be totally ground down by the craziness of the place, descending to the point where you didn't care. Otherwise, a patient you could actually help get out alive might be lost. Even a car with three wheels can be made to ferry a very sick patient from the doomed to the spared. And sometimes along the way, you could even learn a little about yourself.

———

It was the worry and sweetness in her face that moved me most when I first saw Grace O. on morning hospital rounds. She had been admitted from Accident and Emergency just a few hours earlier for shortness of breath and dry cough. Twenty-five years old and a low-level employee in the Ministry of Health, she had never been sick before. Grace's arrival in the female medical ward wasn't very auspicious from the start: it took me and my team several minutes before we could even find her. It was a common problem at Marina, often with fatal results.

More than a few patients admitted to Marina were overlooked, lost in the hospital's haphazard admissions process. First, it was often unclear which team of residents was responsible for a new admission. Not infrequently, a newly admitted patient wouldn't be seen by a doctor for several days. The nurses would duly check the vital signs and write their nursing notes, but it rarely occurred to them to wonder why there were no medical orders in the chart beyond those written in the emergency room, or why a doctor hadn't seen the patient subsequently.

Sometimes the nurses wouldn't call a doctor until the neglected patient died. On my very first day at Morning Report, the morning meeting of all the teams, the head of medicine lambasted a hapless resident who hadn't seen a patient admitted to his team for five days, until the patient, a thirty-two-year-old woman with pneumonia and AIDS, was found dead. He had no excuse—his team had just overlooked her. Too often the residents, never eager to increase their workload, weren't too curious about locating new admissions. I was always paranoid about this happening to my team.

Even if newly admitted patients were on the list to be seen on morning rounds, finding them was often a challenge, because many times the patients didn't have any wrist IDs. Of course, they were supposed to, and probably somewhere in the hospital was a locked closet full of new ID bracelets, which someone had hidden so they wouldn't run out of them—at Marina, the logic made perfect sense—just as most staff wouldn't order new supplies or drugs until they had run out. The nurses rarely kept an updated census of who was where on the ward, so at the start of rounds my resident, intern, and students would fan through the cubicles, going from bed to bed, asking patients if they were so-and-so. If a new patient was severely demented or unconscious—a common occurrence—they would ask the patient's neighbor.

Grace was on our list of new admissions, but we didn't know which of the ward's five cubicles she was in. After the usual wild goose chase, we finally found her in a far corner of the last cubicle, desperately panting into her oxygen mask. She barely had the strength to signal to the resident when he shouted out her name to the twelve denizens of the overcrowded cubicle. But she still was able to smile and weakly extend her hand when I introduced myself. She tried to remove her oxygen mask to greet me, but I gently stayed her hand. Grace was still wearing her street clothes, which, with her slight frame, concealed whatever wasting she might have had. She appeared very worried, as if she didn't understand what was happening to her. After introducing myself, I stepped back to the foot of the bed to review her chart.

The Accident and Emergency note seemed familiar in its litany of Grace's symptoms: HIV status unknown, no prior illnesses, several weeks of cough and shortness of breath, junky-sounding lungs, chest X-ray showing an extensive pneumonia, the obligatory first dose of intravenous antibiotics, and—what especially caught my attention—a pulse oximetry reading of 65 percent. The pulse oximeter—a simple contraption with a clothes-pin-like monitor that's clipped onto the patient's finger—is an easy way to measure at bedside the amount of oxygen in the blood. It should normally be in the upper 90 percent range, and when it dips below that, especially as low as Grace's, it means that the lungs can't oxygenate the blood, and the tissues—the brain, the heart, the kidneys—are in jeopardy of failing. I asked one of the medical students to recheck it.

"Do we have an HIV test?"

"Yes, it's positive," my resident replied.

"Does she know?" I glanced over my shoulder to be sure Grace couldn't hear us. She was smiling at the hapless student trying to check her pulse ox.

"I don't know," the resident said.

Although Botswana had an "opt-out" policy regarding HIV testing— you're supposed to tell the patient you're going to do an HIV test, and if he doesn't scream bloody murder and refuse, you do it—it was doubtful that anyone had asked Grace for permission to test her. In the chaos of Accident and Emergency, such niceties were often dispensed with.

"Seventy percent," chirped the medical student. Not good, especially since she was already on oxygen. Such a low oxygen level in the blood—hypoxemia—meant that Grace was on the edge of the precipice, her vital organs starving for oxygen.

"Check your own pulse ox, to see if the machine is working." A cardinal rule in medicine: if you don't like a lab result, repeat it until you get one you like. Although I was grasping at straws, the equipment at Marina was never routinely recalibrated and our machine could possibly be on the blink. Grace smiled as the student awkwardly applied the device to his index finger. The display read out 99 percent. I turned back to our patient. Naturally—as if not doing it would be wrong—I gently held her hand.

"How are you feeling? Do you feel better, worse, or the same since you got here?" I always liked patients to roughly grade their symptoms, hoping they'd say "better."

"I think . . . the same." Then a brief outburst of coughing followed by even more rapid respirations.

Not bothering to ask about any other symptoms—it was doubtful if she could even speak in full sentences—I set about doing a brief exam. Except for rapid breathing and fast heart rate, the only other thing I found was some thrush in her mouth, a sign that Grace's immune system was very weak. On the other side of the bed, the other three medical students were playing with the pulse ox machine, checking their oxygen saturations. I shot them a perturbed look, and they scampered to the foot of the bed, with the intern and resident. I held Grace's hand again.

"Grace, your HIV test came back positive." I had always favored the direct approach, especially when the patient was very sick and I had little time to spare. She nodded her understanding. I didn't see any sense in asking her if she already knew or suspected. Besides, this was Botswana, and HIV wasn't unusual.

"You have a very bad pneumonia, and we're going to give you antibiotics, which should help you feel better." More nodding of understanding.

"And when you're better, we'll start you on HIV treatment. There's every hope you'll get better." She squeezed my hand. I then half-wished I hadn't given her hope, fearful of provoking the indifferent fates. "Just try to rest, and keep your oxygen on all the time, OK?" Another nod. She seemed to want to talk, but was too preoccupied with breathing. I went back to the team at the foot of the bed to map out a plan.

"Do we have a chest X-ray?" Although the Accident and Emergency doctor had noted bilateral infiltrates on the chest X-ray, it always helped to clarify a patient in your mind by looking at it yourself. The students set to work, and started to check under the corners of her mattress for the X-ray—it was the standard place for a patient's X-rays to be kept.

"There wasn't any film to print it out," the resident reported. Marina's radiology department was regularly plagued with shortages of X-ray film. Presumably the Accident and Emergency doctor had looked at the computer image. Although they were always very busy, the emergency room doctors usually didn't make things up, and their reports could be believed.

"OK, guys, what do you think is going on with her? She's HIV, in respiratory distress, and has diffuse bilateral infiltrates. Dry cough and pulse ox in the seventies." Although always tempted to take total control and bark out treatment orders so I could move rounds forward, I tried to include my team in therapeutic decisions—after all, I was a lecturer in the medical school. Since it seemed to be a fairly straightforward case, I first questioned the medical students, who proffered diagnoses of PCP, TB, and bacterial pneumonia. The intern and resident agreed, as did I.

"In the States, this patient would have had a bronchoscopy in the emergency room before she even hit the ward, and the pathologists would be reading it just now and would tell us the diagnosis before lunch." Bronchoscopy involved sedating the patient and putting a flexible scope down the trachea and lungs, to get specimens for pathology. But bronchoscopies weren't routinely done at Marina, and if they were, there was a long waiting list, often extending to many months. Furthermore, the specimens would have to be sent to South Africa, the report returning months later. Thus, doctors had to base their treatment on pure clinical suspicion.

"This sounds a lot like PCP and not TB," I continued, more thinking out loud than trying to educate my team. "TB usually doesn't cause such profound respiratory distress with this degree of hypoxemia, at least up to the very end." I made sure Grace didn't hear "up to the very end." By then the resident was already writing orders for treatment of her presumed AIDS pneumonia. "She needs to be moved to HDU"—the high-dependency unit, the cubicle closest to the nursing station—"and I want someone to check on her later today before you knock off. Let me know if she's worse." As my team moved on to the next admission, I turned and gave Grace a thumbs-up. She waved and smiled. I tried not to think any more about her, fearful that my desire for her to be spared might jinx her chances.

The next new admission on our list was in the same cubicle, directly across from Grace. Charity K., a forty-year-old housekeeper, was also admitted from Accident and Emergency with pneumonia, and was also in respiratory distress. Unlike Grace, Charity had been diagnosed HIV-positive two years ago during her second bout of TB, but, according to the admission note, she had "defaulted" on ARV therapy a year ago. I always cringed at the word, since it was loaded with self-righteous judgement, as if the patient was at fault and was getting what she deserved.

"We doctors love to blame the patient," I often held forth to the residents and medical students. "If they smoke, they deserve lung cancer; if they're fat, they deserve their diabetes; if they have unprotected sex, they deserve HIV. It's as if we let ourselves off the hook when we can blame the patient and don't feel we should be accountable for their care. As a certain itinerant Galilean rabbi said two thousand years ago, let him among us without sin cast the first stone."

So, Charity was a defaulter, whatever the hell that meant. She'd been having several weeks of fevers, night sweats, and cough. According to the Accident and Emergency note, she was in "acute respiratory failure," with very labored breathing. Her initial pulse ox in the emergency room was 68 percent, barely above Grace's.

"We thought we'd have to intubate her," my intern reported as I perused the admission note, "but her chest X-ray showed a large pneumothorax"—a collapsed lung—"and she calmed down once we put in a chest tube, and her pulse ox went to 88 percent." Almost at the magic 90 percent mark. Sure enough, exiting the left side of her chest was a chest tube hooked up to a plastic bottle. Her lung had re-expanded, and intubation had been averted. One of the medical students had fished her chest X-ray from under a corner of her mattress and was holding it up to the ceiling light, squinting to read it. I didn't bother to ask how or why we had Charity's X-ray from Accident and Emergency when Grace's couldn't be printed out because of lack of film—I just would have received shrugs. I grabbed the X-ray from the student and held it towards the window. The X-ray viewing box by the nursing station had been out of order forever. I handed the film over to the other students, asking them what they saw. They huddled around the X-ray and quickly picked up the abnormalities—upper- and lower-lobe pneumonia of the right lung, which had several large cavities. Most of the students here were eager to learn, but once they became Marina interns and residents, their only concern was to survive the busy on-call nights.

Charity looked sick—weak, malnourished, and slightly pulling for air—but she could speak in complete sentences. She also looked slightly worried, but there was less fear and foreboding compared with Grace. It was almost as if Charity didn't care whether she lived or died. Without prompting, one of the students rechecked her pulse ox—98 percent. Bingo!

Whereas Grace smelled more like PCP, everything in Charity's case—the productive cough, her history of recurrent TB, and a chest-X-ray showing a collapsed lung and large cavities—screamed TB. My doctors had seen a lot more disease here than I had, and I turned to my intern and resident and asked them what we should treat her with. We all agreed on ATT—anti-TB therapy—plus a standard antibiotic for possible bacterial pneumonia. But then, another problem.

"I left my daughter alone. There is no one to look after her."

"How old is she?" Children here grow up fast, and maybe Charity's child was at least an adolescent.

"She is four." Great, I thought to myself. A four-year-old at home alone.

"Isn't there any family you can call?" Nope, there was none. The partner had left her years ago, presumably when she first tested positive. There was an aunt in Francistown, but that was a three-hour drive away. I looked helplessly to my resident.

"We will ask the social worker to see the girl," he replied. What little safety net existed here was largely provided by the social workers. I had never seen any of them on the wards—their offices were somewhere in the large administration building—but sometimes they were able to help with such things. Then, another straw to grasp at.

"Shouldn't a TB nurse see the daughter? Maybe she can help with her." One thing Botswana had going for it was a robust TB program. Even non-citizens, including illegal immigrants, could get ATT for their TB. And the TB nurses actually visited families exposed to TB and tested them. There was a strong sense of community here, and it was possible that the TB nurse, seeing a four-year-old girl alone because her mother was in Marina, might be able to marshal an interim plan to look after the child. My resident said he'd call the TB people after rounds. Just then, another possible solution struck me.

"Can you call your aunt in Francistown to ask her to come look after your daughter?"

"I don't have airtime." For the poor, the cellphone companies demanded prepayment. I pulled my cellphone out and handed it to her.

"Call her, now." We stood around the bed as she spoke to her aunt in Setswana. She paused and looked up. "She cannot afford the bus to come." I turned to my team.

"How much is bus fare from Francistown?" Around thirty pula. I pulled out my folded bills, peeled off a two hundred pula note, and held it in front of Charity. After bus fare, there was enough to feed the aunt and the child for a week. I really hated—*loathed*—playing the role of the rich, beneficent white man, but I needed to tick off at least one serious problem on my list. And if the cost of actually getting something done was two hundred pula, so be it.

"Tell your aunt there's two hundred pula waiting for her if she gets on the next bus here and looks after your daughter." More back and forth in Setswana before ending the call. She handed the phone back to me.

"She will come." Praise the Lord. I handed over the two hundred pula. "But I still want the social worker and TB people involved," I told my resident. But before moving on to the next patient, an important detail.

"Has your daughter been tested for HIV?" It was very possible that Charity was infected when she was pregnant. An embarrassed look of shame. Even if the four-year-old seemed to be well, she could still be infected and might crash and burn later.

"Well, when you're better and out of here, you really must get her tested. It's important!" A nod of understanding.

Grace and Charity, however, weren't the sickest patients on our service—we had several who were comatose or so wasted that their chances of survival were practically nil. But both of them had just a single problem—pneumonia—which made their management easier. Too many of our patients were too far gone, with multiple organ systems profoundly affected, and even if they were in a large American medical center, their conditions would have been a major challenge. Because Marina's myriad deficiencies made orderly evaluation impossible, these patients usually were doomed to die. If they did survive, it often was due to the remarkable reparative ability of the body, and not anything that we doctors could do. But we might be able to help Grace and Charity, so that they could eventually be started on ARVs, with all the promise they entailed.

Over the next few days, Grace and Charity were in a holding pattern, no better and no worse. Grace's pulse ox barely reached 80 percent, and it hurt just to look at her as she devoted her entire being to breathing. But she always managed a smile on rounds. Charity was still weak and slightly breathless. Her aunt had arrived, and, according to the nurses' notes, she wanted to be counselled about her niece's condition—it was always a good sign when the family wished to be included. I wasn't alarmed at their lack of progress: patience is necessary in such cases. Each day, as I did for every patient, I checked the medication sheets to be sure they were actually getting their antibiotics—frequently, medicines wouldn't be given, for reasons not known even to God. But simply because the medication box had been ticked off by the nurse was no guarantee: it was not uncommon that drugs marked as given actually weren't.

By the end of the first week, Charity was perking up. She no longer had fevers, and her respirations were no longer labored. She was walking to the ward's bathroom, and her chest tube had been removed. Her sputum specimen for TB testing was lost by the lab—a common occurrence—and the ward subsequently had a shortage of plastic cups for collecting another specimen. But I felt confident of the diagnosis of TB and had no problem consigning her to an obligatory six-month treatment as an outpatient.

Grace, on the other hand, was no better. Still tugging for air, she hadn't even changed out of her street clothes, probably because the effort would have been too much for her. It wasn't unusual for PCP to take a week or so before responding to treatment, but what if she didn't have PCP and had something else? What if she, too, had TB? The echocardiogram we'd ordered returned normal, making heart problems unlikely, and there was no evidence of blood clots in her lungs causing her breathlessness. I still hadn't seen her admission chest X-ray, despite my asking for it daily on rounds. By the beginning of the second week, I was out of patience.

"All right, if we can't find her X-ray, then we need to repeat it. We're treating a pneumonia without even knowing what the chest X-ray looks like." I was out of Grace's earshot, so she didn't hear the frustration in my voice.

"There's no portable oxygen to take her to X-ray." My resident's reply was matter-of-fact. Faced daily with the multiple shortages and other lapses in care at Marina, his equanimity was remarkable. He cared about his patients, but accepted the deficiencies here. And the portable X-ray machine had been out of commission for over a year.

When I went over to Grace, she was barely able to speak, and for the first time she didn't smile at me. She looked even more worried than before, and small beads of perspiration coated her head. Her blouse was moist from perspiration. Her pulse ox clocked in at 67 percent.

"Grace, I think there's a possibility that you might have TB, so we're going to start TB medicine, but still continue your other antibiotics." As on my prior visits, I held her hand and looked straight into her eyes. She nodded her agreement. I quickly debated whether to reassure her, as I'd done on every other visit.

"Just hang in there. It will be fine." Not to reassure her might have frightened her even more. Away from the bed, I shared with the team another ominous possibility, which I was loath to give words to. So loath that I actually whispered to my team.

"This might be pulmonary KS. She doesn't have any lesions"—I had carefully rechecked her skin and mouth the day before—"but that doesn't mean anything." Usually, patients with lung Kaposi's had at least a few purplish spots on their skin or in their mouths, but the absence of such lesions was no guarantee that the lungs weren't riddled with the cancer. In Marina, pulmonary KS was usually fatal—the patient suffocated to death. ARVs and chemotherapy were "Hail Mary passes" that might help, but the side effects often limited their use, especially in patients who were wasting away. But except for her lungs, Grace was in fairly good shape—she wasn't a bedridden skeleton with respiratory failure, like so many patients here. The only way to diagnose lung KS was by bronchoscopy, which would show reddish-purple spots studding the bronchial tree—no need to send specimens to South Africa. Not only was urgent bronchoscopy difficult to get, but her condition made it very risky—she could have a respiratory arrest during the procedure. We would have to have an ICU bed available if she crashed during it. Against the odds, I decided to try the "Hail Mary pass."

First, I had to see if we could get her bronched. The hospital specialist who did them was Dr. Yak, a quiet and reserved Chinese doctor of indeterminate age who had been at Marina for a long time, maybe forever. We never really had much interaction but he was always pleasant and courteous. At Morning Report, he would frequently doze off. But I wasn't surprised when, after explaining Grace's case with him, he readily agreed to scope her the next morning, as long as one of the team doctors was there. He even said he'd intubate her if she arrested during the procedure. I vowed to myself never again to be annoyed if he started snoring during a resident's presentation.

Arranging an ICU bed if she tanked during the procedure would be a big problem. ICU had always been a fiefdom unto itself, run by anesthesiologists and the occasional intensivist on duty. There was always ambiguity about who was really in charge of a patient who ended up in ICU—ward specialists like me would follow our patients transferred there, but we'd never manage the ventilator settings or the various cardiac drugs being given. Many patients in the place were comatose, hooked up to breathing machines, with every orifice probed or tubed. During my first stint in Botswana, I had visited a very sad patient for a friend of mine—his pregnant housekeeper had suffered a catastrophic stroke, and had been comatose, in a vegetative state for over a month. I asked one of the ICU nurses if anyone had discussed with the family the option of disconnecting all of the machines and tubes, to give her a semblance of dignity as she died. The nurse seemed shocked that I would even suggest such a thing. "*Oh no*, doctor, in Botswana we let patients die a *natural* death." Yes, ICU was an alternative universe of sorts. I wasn't optimistic as I carefully discussed Grace's case with the Chinese doctor on duty in ICU. Her verdict, while astonishing, was what I'd expected.

"*She have the AIDS!* We no take patient with the AIDS!" Annoyance –hostility—that I'd dare disturb her with such a thing. Time and again, we'd hear at Morning Report how patients who needed ICU care were denied entry either because they were HIV-positive or because their T-cell counts were very low. The head of medicine would quietly sit through such reports and check messages on her BlackBerry, because she knew that confronting the ICU was a losing proposition. But the sweeping ignorance about HIV infection at this late date still amazed me. Even some of the surgeons were leery of operating on HIV patients, citing "poor wound healing" and other such rubbish, which had been debunked over twenty years previously. Although I wanted to tell the ICU doctor to pull her clueless head out of her sorry ass and come into the 21st century, I persisted politely, emphasizing how Grace looked otherwise well nourished, and how it was possible that she might not need a bed anyway. Several times I noted how diagnosing KS and then treating it with chemotherapy was her only chance at this point. But then the ultimate brush-off, the pronouncement for which there was no appeal.

"We full. ICU full. We no have beds." It was the standard ICU response—cop-out—for keeping out new patients. It was far easier to care for the comatose patients occupying the beds, who were essentially on autopilot. I asked the ICU doctor to stop by the ward and put a note in Grace's chart. She put the phone down on me.

Fortunately, I hadn't told Grace about my plans for bronchoscopy, as I didn't want to get her hopes up. I phoned Dr. Yak with the bad news, and he said he stood ready to help in the future.

That afternoon, I stopped by the female ward, ostensibly to document in Grace's chart my failed attempt at bronchoscopy, but really to see how she was doing. Visiting hours were in full swing, and the cubicles were crammed with friends and family at the bedsides. Some were bathing loved ones, emptying urinals, changing the bed, or bringing in extra food and juice. Some of the beds were circled with people, many praying out loud in Setswana, even singing hymns. Bibles were waved about in the air, hands outstretched to Heaven. Sometimes the prayers were shouted out, often stridently, as if they were casting out demons, or—I feared—castigating the patient for his or her alleged sinfulness and insisting on the need to repent.

There were no visitors at Grace's bedside—her only family was an older sister in the States, who couldn't be reached despite our best attempts. Oblivious to the cacophony around her, she was asleep, although still with rapid and labored breathing. For the umpteenth time I racked my brain for what we might be missing. We were treating PCP and TB. Heart problems and lung clots had been ruled out. Maybe it was a rare disease like scleroderma, but she had no other evidence for it. KS seemed the most likely cause, but we couldn't diagnose it, at least at Marina.

The next morning on rounds, after little over a week at Marina, Charity was on the launching pad, ready to be discharged home. Many times we'd send our sickest patients home to die, or we'd just give up on trying to diagnose what was wrong with them and would discharge them with an appointment in the outpatient clinic, usually months later, where nothing would be done anyway, assuming they survived until then. A "clean," clear-cut discharge was always savored. Charity was no longer short of breath, and except for malnourishment, she looked well. She said her aunt would stay with her until she was stronger. She fished around in her purse and produced a 200 pula bill, which she handed to me.

"My employer"—a few days earlier I learned she worked for the Turkish consul—"said I should give this back to you. He has taken care of my auntie and daughter." I knew the man peripherally. He was a Botswana story if ever there was one, having been a close friend and advisor of Sir Seretse and Lady Ruth Khama, until his political enemies ruthlessly defanged him. Well into his eighties, Mohammed did not suffer fools, and his tongue was a rapier on which many fools had been impaled. But he took care of "his people," such as Charity. My initial impulse was to tell her to keep the two hundred, but that would have insulted her. I thanked her for returning it. But before we said goodbye, I once again had to make sure she finally got HIV treatment.

"Charity, you must get HIV treatment as soon as possible. You almost died, and how would that have helped your daughter? And you have to get her tested for HIV! Please go to the nearest clinic and demand that you get treated and your daughter gets tested. Give them your discharge paper that the resident will give you in a bit. Do you understand?" I couldn't tell from her face whether she fully understood, or even cared. I turned to my team, who were probably bracing themselves to hear yet again my standard tirade for such patients.

"Guys!!! You *must*—I repeat, *must*—review with her where to go for her ARVs. Find out which clinic is nearest. And I want her discharge summary to clearly indicate that she must—I repeat, *must*—be started on ARVs as soon as possible! Put down my name and number for them to call if they have to. I want the ARV clinic to have a platinum-engraved invitation to start her on ARVs." I would always do everything short of jumping onto the bed and doing a vivid fan dance to impress upon my team how they needed to be sure that patients like Charity weren't discharged with vague instructions, only to fall through the cracks once again.

"We will do it," my resident replied. I waved goodbye to Charity, feeling I'd done all I could do. The rest was up to her.

Grace was awake, and she smiled as I approached her bed. She looked worse, if that was possible. Her breathing was even more labored, and her heart rate was 180 per minute, up from her prior 130 rate. Her clothes were soaked with perspiration. I went through the motions of checking her heart and lungs. I waved away the medical student who had brought the pulse ox machine to the bed. I gently held her hand.

"Grace, we're going to give you a medicine called morphine. It will relax you and help your breathing." We had nothing more to offer. We wouldn't knock out her respiratory drive, but the morphine would hopefully reduce her anxiety and discomfort. "It should make you feel better." No further promises of recovery, no other words of reassurance. We had to make sure Grace died with a minimum of distress. She said nothing—every ounce of energy was now concentrated on trying to take the next breath—but she smiled again.

At a safe distance, I discussed with the team our plan for regular injections of morphine. They understood my reasoning, but I wanted to be sure that they were comfortable with these last rites that we were about to administer. Unanimous nods of agreement.

Later that afternoon, I stopped by to see how she was doing. I told myself that my visit was purely clinical—to be sure the morphine was keeping her comfortable—and not one of my misguided, self-indulgent attempts to provide "emotional support" to a dying patient. Many times in the past, I had had similar urges with other patients whose suffering and impending demise had moved me. But I had come to realize that such gestures of seeming compassion were largely for my own benefit, and not for the patient. For many patients who realize they're dying, their focus changes—they're somewhere else that's beyond the understanding of those of us still living. They don't need new friends or well-meaning attempts at compassion. Twenty years ago, at St Clare's, I held lots of hands. But now I knew that it had been meaningful to me only because I thought it was meaningful to my patients, when most of the time it wasn't.

Grace was sleeping, snowed under by the morphine. Gazing dumbly at her, I felt a profound sense of loss, of free-floating sadness. I resisted the urge to hold her hand one last time.

The next morning on rounds, I learned that Grace had died the previous evening. I thought about her for several days afterwards. Not so much about whether we had missed something treatable—we did the best we could. Rather, my thoughts centered on an important question which had bothered me ever since I first came to Botswana, over thirteen years previously. It was that finger-to-the-heart question put to me by the cosmopolitan cardiothoracic surgeon at my going-away dinner in New York in 2002, right before I left for Botswana. He had questioned my altruism in going to Africa, and suggested that Africans viewed suffering differently from the way we did.

Over the years in Botswana, the surgeon's words would resurface. At the time, I'd thought to myself, "What an arrogant, self-centered prick! What does he know about suffering, let alone suffering from AIDS in Africa?" But now, I wasn't so sure. Maybe he was right. On one hand, at places like Marina there was never any urgency about anything—if a patient died, that was fine; if she lived, that was fine, too. Some patients like Charity appeared not to care whether they lived or died, even if thrown the life raft of ARVs. But then there were patients like Grace, who seemed worried about leaving this world. And for anyone who has ever stood at the graveside of a funeral here, with a light rain pattering down and family and friends singing hymns of unspeakable beauty and sadness, such an experience is never forgotten. Africans do not suffer differently.

Maybe if I had told my dinner companion many years ago that I was going to Botswana for a new adventure, for my own "selfish" reasons, he might have approved. As my years here rolled by, I realized that the right answer to his query would have been that I was going to Africa to know myself better, to try to save myself.

In *Heart of Darkness*, his amazing journey into the abyss of mankind's inner darkness, Joseph Conrad wrote, "Before the Congo, I was a mere animal." Yes, Africa does that to you, even a much tamer place like Botswana. Perhaps I could say that before Botswana, I was merely a clueless doctor who thought that compassion was as easy as holding the hand of a patient dying from AIDS.

Morning Report was many things, but it was rarely dull. Interesting, exasperating, depressing, inspiring, but never boring. I would always attend with a sense of expectation and dread, wondering what would be the latest amazing case, or mismanagement atrocity, or sad story. Often it would be all three in one. Sometimes, there would even be stories of rescuing a patient from the abyss. Morning Report was a bird's-eye view of the harrowing world of Princess Marina Hospital.

Every weekday morning at 7:30, all of the medical teams gathered to discuss new admissions, present journal articles, and hear the latest announcements. The idea was to improve patient care and further doctor education. All residents and interns on the medical wards were required to attend, as well as the medical students assigned to the medicine rotation. Specialists supervising the six medical teams on the wards were also expected to be present, but often many wouldn't. I'd always go, even if I didn't have ward duty at the time.

The meeting was held in a small conference room in the male medical ward. Barely the size of a bedroom, it accommodated up to several dozen people, often more. Most of the year, the room was very hot, despite the two desultory ceiling fans wobbling overhead.

The chairs crammed into the room were very, very old. The hierarchy in seating was informal, but the students—sometimes up to fifteen or so—always sat at the back, often sharing chairs. From the outset, I had staked out a comfortable chair with arms and a soft cushion, right in the front.

Morning Report's format was pretty standard—it probably hadn't changed for over a generation. One or two doctors from the team on call the night before would present one or two of the dozen or so patients they'd admitted. Unless a resident had garroted a patient in bed, any errors, however egregious, were largely passed over. The interns and residents presented clinical mishaps as a matter of course—screw-ups that in the States would have resulted in lost medical licenses, major sanctions against hospitals, and multi-million-dollar lawsuits. But Morning Report wasn't just a depressing litany of the doomed. Some patients were actually helped. That was the beauty of Morning Report: you never knew whether the next case was going to end up in the morgue, or take up his bed and walk out of hospital alive, a triumph of medical care.

A seventeen-year-old herd boy was admitted for severe pneumonia with respiratory failure, and tested HIV-positive. His chest X-ray was a total "white-out"—his lungs were drowning—and he needed to be put on a breathing machine as soon as possible. But the ICU doctor refused to accept him because he was HIV-positive. Medical futility, they said, and, what is more, they first wanted to know the boy's T-cell count before accepting him into ICU, never mind it would take over a week to get it back. You would have thought it was 1988. He probably could have been saved with proper ICU intervention, but he died on the ward a couple of hours later.

A fifteen-year-old herd boy was brought in comatose and foaming at the mouth, reeking of insecticide. His friend said he'd been messing around with some plant fertilizer before he got sick. We'd see lots of such cases. The intern knew what to do—give industrial doses of atropine repeatedly—and the boy gradually woke up by the morning, eventually to go home and resume herding his goats or cows.

A fifty year-old woman had gone to a traditional healer for her hemorrhoids. He told her to drink thirty gallons of water to purify her system. She did—a veritable triumph of the will—and the resulting water intoxication swelled up her brain. She was brought in over the weekend, seizing and comatose. She made it to ICU, where she was intubated and sedated. By Monday morning, she was off the breathing machine, awake and alert, complaining about her hemorrhoids.

A twelve-year-old boy, unresponsive after being electrocuted by a downed power line, was rushed to Accident and Emergency, where he died from a lethal heart arrhythmia, because the A&E's defibrillator was broken, as was the one they rushed from the ICU. This case actually made it into some of the newspapers, but nothing came of it.

A twenty-year-old woman came in with heart failure—not your grandmother's type of heart failure, but heart failure due to damaged, rotten heart valves from remote rheumatic fever. She also had a serious infection of her valves, which the on-call resident treated with broad-spectrum antibiotics. After two weeks, she was stable and was transferred to South Africa for successful valve replacement.

Sometimes at Morning Report, the malpractice had started outside Marina, before the patient was admitted. A young woman, spared from AIDS several years earlier—her ARVs had boosted her T-cells to 540—had had a long history of severe sulfa allergy. Her outpatient medical cards were plastered with allergy alerts. But some careless doctor in one of the local clinics went ahead and gave her a sulfa antibiotic for a bladder infection. She developed a severe reaction and essentially sloughed off most of her skin. The resident presenting the case showed a picture of her that he had taken with his cellphone: pretty grisly, like a serious burn patient. Blood infection and kidney failure ensued, but the kidney team fobbed off the need for urgent dialysis. She died before she could be transferred to one of the private hospitals for dialysis.

And so on, day after day. For cases of the doomed, the reaction of everyone at Morning Report was remarkable for the total lack of reaction. Even the successes didn't elicit elation. Sometimes for a particularly sad case, there might be a tinge of regret in the resident's presentation. But there was never any sense that these things should not be allowed to happen, or that we needed to find ways to prevent them from happening again.

Morning Report also highlighted the major, recurrent shortages and stock-outs of even the most basic medications and supplies. For several months, blood electrolytes—sodium, potassium—couldn't be done because the lab had run out of necessary reagents. On a recurring basis, for months at a time, contrast CT scans couldn't be done because radiology had run out of the special syringes needed to inject the contrast dye. Stock-outs of crucial intravenous fluids were common—trying to treat diabetic ketoacidosis without normal saline or Ringer's solution was akin to driving a car in Gaborone without brakes, and blindfolded, to boot. The blood bank regularly had no blood in stock, and patients' family members were often asked to donate units in the hope that their blood types were compatible with their loved ones. If not, the patient was just out of luck, and would often die from anemia. And stock-outs of common antibiotics barely merited mentioning. It was just accepted as the way it was. It really was difficult to hold the interns and residents to higher standards of care when the entire system screamed that it didn't care. Botswana had the money—it was a "middle-income" country—but sometimes you would think you were in Sudan or Chad.

As we doctors liked to say, the "pathology" presented at Morning Report was truly extraordinary, with diseases I had previously only read about. Because trying to manage patients expeditiously was impossible, you'd often get to see the gruesome natural history of untreated lung cancer or kidney obstruction or a host of other conditions that in the States would never have been allowed to progress to such advanced stages. It was like seeing diseases play themselves out in the 18th century.

Most of the time, the interns and residents practiced cookbook medicine, following simple, one-size-fits-all steps in diagnosis and treatment. It was tough to blame them, when they regularly had to admit up to a dozen very sick patients every night. And cookbook medicine worked up to a point—many a patient had been saved by following simple ABCs. But as a lecturer, I would always exhort them to "think outside the box," to consider alternative diagnoses and not just the obvious ones. Simply because a patient had wheezing didn't mean her shortness of breath was due to asthma—she could have heart failure, or a blood clot in her lungs, or a blockage of her upper airway.

Finally, Morning Report was never short of bizarre announcements and news. For example, one day the Chief of Medicine reported that the Ministry of Health had arranged for fifty Chinese doctors to come here. The only problem was that they were caught in the bureaucratic morass known as the Health Professions Council. Visiting their offices every year to renew your medical license was an exercise in Zen Buddhist patience. Usually it took at least three visits before their computer system and massive paper files jived and finally regurgitated your renewal. So, we had 50 Chinese doctors in limbo. The Chief of Medicine said she didn't know exactly where they were right then, since they had been waiting for many weeks for their licenses. I had visions of Chinese doctors touring the Okavango Delta, taking tens of thousands of pictures of wild animals. I decided to be naughty and asked her if any of them spoke English—we already had several Cuban doctors who spoke varying degrees of "Spanglish," usually more Spanish than English. She sheepishly replied that they did not. But in fairness to the Chinese, they were usually very proficient in languages, so it wouldn't have surprised me if they eventually learned Setswana rather than English.

━━━━━

In all my years in Botswana, I had never before been asked to fill out an insurance form for a patient. But a year into my job at the medical school, the head of Marina's medicine department asked me to help a patient with his insurance form. She said I'd been the ward specialist when he was an inpatient four months earlier.

Almost all my patients were under government care, in public clinics or hospitals. True, some of them might have had health insurance, entitling them to be admitted to one of the two private hospitals in Gaborone, but if they were really sick, they'd eventually reach the maximum limit of their insurance coverage. When that happened, they were immediately shipped off to Marina. It didn't matter how sick or unstable a patient was—when the money ran out, they were kicked over to Marina. The private hospitals were newer, perhaps a tad cleaner, although Marina was usually tidy enough. But if affluent Batswana or we expatriates ever had a serious problem—a heart attack, stroke, or whatever—we'd all head to one of the major hospitals in Johannesburg, gambling that it'd be better to be shipped several hundred miles away rather than risk it in Gaborone. MRI, the major medical transport company, had always done a brisk business.

Gaborone Private Hospital had been on the scene for decades, managed over the years by too many private companies to count— finances were always a problem. Bokamoso Hospital, built a few years after my first stint in Botswana, was supposed to be the pre-eminent medical center in sub-Saharan Africa, to which even patients from neighboring South Africa would be referred. Several of Botswana's big insurance companies had formed a consortium to finance Bokamoso's construction, and a prominent medical center in the west had been retained to staff it with the best specialists in the world. But as often happens here, things went pear-shaped—thinking they were too important to follow the rules, the medical center allegedly refused to meet certain government requirements and pulled out—and Bokamoso never achieved the exalted promise of its inception. Many people made a lot of money on this project, including a legion of consultants, many American. And you didn't even want to think about the small fortunes more than a few people made from all the backhanders such a massive project would spawn.

In her text message about the insurance form, the head of medicine had included the patient's name—it would have been a miracle if I had recognized it, which I didn't. I texted back to ask her to tell the patient to meet me the next day at 2 p.m. in the male medical ward, when I was sure I'd be finished with ward rounds.

The next afternoon, the patient showed up on time, along with his girlfriend. Themba G. definitely looked familiar—his was the sort of face you'd remember: youthful, pleasant, slightly daft, and totally clueless, almost juvenile despite his thirty-six years. He seemed to have gained weight since I last saw him, almost to the point that he no longer looked drawn and wasted. He seemed happy to see me—I was the man who could unlock some money from his insurance policy, a standard disability arrangement. A quick review of the discharge summary he brought from his hospitalization four months ago jogged my memory. It had been a typical case: a young Motswana, never before HIV tested, who had come in with florid symptoms of meningitis, tested HIV-positive, and was diagnosed with cryptococcal meningitis, a fatal AIDS-related fungal infection of the brain. He was lucky to have been in Marina at just the right time—during his stay, there were no stock-outs of fluconazole, a crucial drug to treat his meningitis—and he woke up from his coma and ultimately left the hospital alive.

After reviewing his discharge summary, I asked Themba what medications he was taking. He produced his bottle of Atripla, the first-line ARV regimen here, plus cotrimoxazole, a once-a-day sulfa drug to prevent serious lung infections due to AIDS.

"Where's your fluconazole?" I asked. A blank look. For someone like Themba, it was absolutely essential that he stay on this powerful antifungal drug until his very low T-cell count increased substantially, which could take many months, maybe even years. His girlfriend, who seemed much more with it, spoke up.

"The clinic didn't have any. We went to another clinic, and there was none." *Holy Mother of God*, this guy was a walking time bomb: the fungus in his brain could quickly gain the upper hand and land him back in Marina with a recurrence of his meningitis. Then a silly question, but I had to ask it anyway.

"Can you afford to pay for it?" There were times when Marina would have brief stock-outs of fluconazole and I would buy a few days' supply for my patients, but there was no way I was going to finance Themba's fluconazole for months and months.

"We can't," the girlfriend replied apologetically. "He can't work. And I earn just enough for food and rent." Fair enough. As I recalled, he had been an electrician at a construction company here, a job that probably had paid good money plus his insurance policy. With the high unemployment, he was lucky his girlfriend had a job.

No fluconazole in a middle-income country where AIDS and its complications were as common as mosquitoes in summer. We were at an impasse—or, rather, Themba was at an impasse, up the Okavango Delta without a paddle, the crocodiles snapping at his flimsy canoe. I was surprised at my reaction, since many of my patients had faced similar situations in the past. I quietly shook my head in despair.

No fluconazole. Disgust and anger welled up inside me. Almost since the beginning of time, Central Medical Stores (CMS), the government agency responsible for ordering and supplying the country's hospitals and clinics with drugs, had been a profoundly dysfunctional, don't-give-a-damn bureaucracy. In 2006, an outside consultancy found egregious deficiencies in the place: animal and human excrement scattered among the storage areas, expired drugs, drugs that were reported to be out of stock but were found hidden away, staff who never did a stock check, and outright graft and corruption. The latter problem culminated in a highly publicized case involving CMS staff, some of whom were sent to prison for defrauding the government of twenty-two million pula. Meanwhile, a patient with serious fungal meningitis went without crucial antibiotics, or a diabetic patient couldn't get insulin, or someone's blood pressure soared because of a shortage of medications.

"Themba, you have to be on the fluconazole so you don't get meningitis again." Blank looks from him, but comprehension from his girlfriend. "You have to go back to the clinics until they give it to you. If there's still no fluconazole, you have to contact your member of parliament and complain high to hell that you're going to die if you don't get it!" Even more mystified looks: the thought of engaging his MP was totally foreign to him.

The form Themba presented was pretty straightforward—I'd done probably thousands in the States. As I filled it out, Themba sat across the table from me and watched intently. When I came to the section about how disabled he was, he fidgeted a bit in his chair, cleared his throat nervously, and leaned forward ever so slightly. His intense interest in which box I ticked confirmed that he wasn't as clueless as he appeared. The questions gave me several options for Themba's disability: temporary or permanent, partial or total.

I didn't dislike Themba—I mean, how can you dislike a guy with AIDS recovering from meningitis who had lost his job and was getting screwed over by whatever cone-heads were responsible for the lack of fluconazole in the clinic pharmacies? But I was only human, and, to me, he seemed to have the fatuous, birdbrained personality that always annoyed the hell out of me, especially whenever I'd try to stay alive driving around the city.

Part of being a doctor has always been not letting your own personal prejudices interfere with the care of your patients, and if Themba happened to be one of the legions of morons on the roads—and he probably was—I wouldn't let that affect my care for him or how I filled out his disability form. Ideally, the goal of HIV treatment should be returning the patient to a normal life. Themba's disability should have been temporary and partial—he looked as if he could do some menial, low-intensity job, probably part-time—and, eventually, he should have improved so he could resume his electrician job. But in Botswana the unemployment rate was 25 percent, higher among recent college graduates. And he didn't have any fluconazole and could possibly end up back in Marina, ultimately with brain damage. In the States, I always gave the patient the benefit of the doubt in such cases. I firmly ticked off "Permanent Total Disability." Themba sat back in the chair. He'd be getting a large sum from the insurance company. I didn't want to think how he would spend it.

"Themba, you need to use any money you get from this for your fluconazole, or else you'll get sick again and probably die."

Another blank look.

"We will do it, doctor. And I will visit my MP to complain"—the firm resolve of a Motswana woman who meant business. At least the girlfriend had some sense. Many clueless Batswana males—not to mention American ones—have been saved by their girlfriends, wives, sisters, mothers, aunts, and grandmothers. Hopefully Themba would have enough sense to let his girlfriend take control.

As I watched the two of them leave with the insurance form, I reflected upon what I had just done. Not the matter of stretching the truth about Themba's disability—I could not have cared less about the ethics of giving him wiggle room so he could get a payout. But I again mulled over whether all of this—the HIV Treatment Programme, indeed any medical intervention at all—was at the end of the day just a zero-sum game. That is, was it possible that every "good" deed—in this case, sparing Themba from death from AIDS—would be counterbalanced by equally bad results? Themba would soon have a lot of money, and he could get drunk and crash his car into a kombi, killing the dozen or so people crammed into it, people who otherwise would have lived if I had not treated his AIDS. Or maybe someday he might achieve a state of grace and eventually father a child who would find the cure for cancer. I'd never know. Besides, it was none of my business.

Some of my cynical friends in Botswana would argue that the National HIV/AIDS Treatment Programme was a zero-sum proposition, that any good or benefit from saving someone from AIDS could very likely result in the saved person eventually causing more harm than good. I would always counter that to be human, we must always err on the side of mercy, of compassionate action. A zero-sum approach was a nihilistic cop-out, an excuse for inaction, for not caring. After taking the calculation of good versus bad outcomes to the tenth or even hundredth decimal point, I wanted to hope that the result would be positive, however minuscule.

But whenever I was on the roads, I would always be on guard for all the Thembas out there.

# Chapter 16

# Outreach, Ten Years Later

Just as Botswana is a country most people have heard about but can't locate on a map, so it's been with the Kalahari Desert, the empty expanse in the western part of the country. The Setswana word for the place means "the great thirst," or another word for it means "a waterless place." The Kalahari wasn't a desert in the sense of endless sand dunes traversed by camel caravans, although it did have camels, imported generations ago from East Africa. Rather, it was dusty, dry bush, populated by warthogs, lizards, birds of prey, lions, and the odd little village such as Hukuntsi, population 4,654, at least according to the 2011 census, and not counting the ubiquitous wild donkeys. Out in the middle of the Kalahari, in the emptiness of western Botswana, Hukuntsi made Molepolole, my first outreach visit, look like a thriving metropolis. Even though it was a small village, it actually had a district hospital, which also served the even smaller villages surrounding it.

Outreach visits to Hukuntsi required a chartered single-propeller plane to ferry me and three or four pediatricians and surgeons to the boondocks. Getting there by air was usually fine, but the return flights often bumped into Botswana's late-day thunderstorms. To gaze on the face of God, fly through one of Botswana's thunderstorms. Once, we hit such turbulence that my glasses flew off and pens leapt out of my shirt pocket, smacking the ceiling. During such moments, I would recall how forty years previously, as a medical student, when I took Allegheny Airlines from Philadelphia to Columbus in their rickety Lockheed Electras, I'd bargain with God to save me from turbulence, promising to become a medical missionary. Of course, after being spared from crashing into the Appalachians, I'd always forget my vow and resume my wicked ways. Now, the joke was that I didn't believe in God anymore and, moreover, I had already become a medical missionary of sorts.

On our outreach visit to Hukuntsi, as we briskly strode to our aircraft, there was the familiar sense of exhilaration and space I had every time I was about to fly to somewhere else, away from boring Gaborone. The cool morning breezes enveloped us, the translucent blue sky welcoming the rising sun. Bounding into the tiny airplane, we crammed into our seats. The male pilot gave us a quick safety briefing—not much to say except that the emergency exit was the small door we had entered by—and he and the co-pilot, an attractive woman as young as her colleague, squeezed past us into the cockpit. Quickly thereafter, the roaring buzz of the single propeller rattled and shook the aircraft on taxiing to the runway, and no sooner did the take-off roll start than we were airborne. The runway beneath us seemed to go on and on before trailing off into bush. Gaborone was soon behind us.

An hour later, our descent into the greater Hukuntsi area was quick—no traffic controllers to put us in a holding pattern. In fact, there was no air traffic at all, except for us, probably the first in weeks. From the air, the village seemed very spread out, with scattered huts and cattle kraals surrounded by bare ground. Having flown on outreach to other villages, I knew that landing was a dicey proposition—the unpaved runways were very short, with the added risk of donkeys, goats, or cows lazing on the landing strip. But our pilots had done this before, and in short order we were piling out of the airplane onto the gravel runway, which was surrounded by barbed-wire fencing. Only one forlorn donkey was grazing just on the other side. In the distance was a petrol station, but we were otherwise out in the country.

The "terminal" was a small one-room building with a few worn chairs and bathrooms, plus two large bathrooms outside, just next to the building. The various city councils throughout the country had a thing about buildings having plenty of bathrooms. The only sign of life was two grounds men, one napping in the shade and the other half-heartedly raking the gravel outside the terminal. There was nothing else, save for a limp wind stocking and a small fuel storage tank. We really were at the ends of the earth.

The hospital vehicle that was supposed to meet us was thirty minutes late. The ten-minute drive afforded us a chance to see Hukuntsi close-up: scattered huts, two gas stations, a discount furniture store, a tiny post office, and two grocery stores. There weren't many people out and about, and those who were stirring seemed laid-back and languid.

The entrance to the Hukuntsi District Hospital said it all. Just outside the front door was a small pond of muddy water from a recent storm, with swarms of mosquitoes buzzing above it. A rusted roof gutter had collapsed, probably long ago, and was dangling directly over the entranceway. Off to the side a goat was resting contentedly on its haunches. We had to circumnavigate the pond, the gutter, and the goat to get in. As we entered, a stray dog roaming the clinic waiting area was being shooed out by an obese nurse, who kindly directed us to the superintendent's office. Even though we had been expected, protocol dictated that our first stop should be the superintendent, to exchange pleasantries. However, the secretary, who was also the hospital telephone operator and janitor, told us that he had "gone out" and wouldn't be back for several hours. As on prior outreach visits, I first headed to the inpatient ward, to make rounds with the doctor there.

Hukuntsi's inpatient medical ward—actually, it also served as the surgery, obstetrics, and gynecology wards as well—was less than half the size of just one of Marina's. The hallway separated the males from the females. Although it was early June, Christmas tinsel still decorated the walls, and at the small nursing station a very tired-appearing artificial Christmas tree held lonely vigil. Dr. Maku, a medical officer from Somalia, was in charge of the whole operation, and he seemed happy to see me.

"Dr. Baxter! You were my teacher at KITSO many years ago! Do you remember me?" Yet another "Baxter protégé," or so it would seem. We set out on our rounds. The understanding with these outreach visits was that the doctors were supposed to consult us on only the more difficult cases. But practically all of the patients here were difficult cases. Unlike Marina, which could have up to a hundred adult patients on its medical wards, the patient census here was very small. The ward nurse joined Dr. Maku and me, and we started with the males. An overpowering odor greeted us.

"He came in two days ago," Dr. Maku introduced the first patient, "and he tested HIV-positive, and we don't know what to do with him. He has bad diarrhea." In a corner, sitting cross-legged on a tattered mattress on the floor, was a malnourished young man, probably in his mid-twenties, who was naked except for a T-shirt which had the Vision 2016 logo on it, with its motto "AIDS-Free Generation." Vision 2016, announced over ten years previously with great fanfare, was Botswana's grand plan to rid the country of new HIV infections by 2016, the fiftieth anniversary of the country's independence. At the time, 2016 seemed like light years into the future, promising plenty of time to get the HIV house in order, but now it was only a few years away. The patient, mattress, and T-shirt were smeared with liquid stool, and he was distractedly rubbing some of it in his straggly hair. Dr. Maku and our nurse seemed unperturbed. I had to give Marina its due: a sight like that wouldn't be tolerated—he would have been hosed down and strapped into bed. The man had the wide glassy-eyed stare of dementia, or worse. It was the sort of stare you'd never forget once you saw it: it was as if he was having a vision of sheer terror, of looking into the abyss.

"What did his spinal tap show?" A fair question, one which a resident at Marina would usually answer before you asked it. Sure, he probably had HIV dementia, but meningitis was the thing to rule out.

"He doesn't have any fever and his neck isn't stiff. I don't think we have any spinal needles."

"We have them," the nurse chimed in, with a slight tinge of impatience.

"Okay then, he really needs a spinal tap as soon as possible. The lack of fever and stiff neck doesn't mean anything. There's a good chance he could have cryptococcal or TB meningitis." Although astonished at Maku's nonchalance, I tried to be as collegial as possible. Alienating the only doctor who stood between this patient and death would accomplish nothing. Maku squirmed and nodded.

Next was a fifty-six year-old man, a policeman, who had been admitted a week ago for a stroke. Sure enough, he couldn't talk or move his right arm or leg. The nurse knew him—they went to the same church—and she said his blood pressure hadn't been controlled for many years.

"He went to the clinic, but they just gave him the same medicines. Some of them were out of stock, but they just gave him the same medicines." Even after twelve years of operation, the HIV/AIDS Treatment Programme was still monopolizing medical resources in the country, at the expense of hypertension, heart disease, and other maladies that affected far more Batswana than HIV did. The patient had an erratic, irregular heart rate—I suspected atrial fibrillation, which probably was the source of the blood clot to his brain. I asked a silly question.

"Did you get an ECG on him? I think he has atrial fibrillation." Nope, no ECG machine—such high-tech equipment was only to be found at Marina.

"OK, this guy needs to go to Marina so he can get a CT scan and ECG." As pathetic as Marina could be, this patient needed to be transferred for what little evaluation we could do there.

A 43-year-old man had come in comatose a few days previously. "We are waiting for the family to arrive to give permission for the spinal tap. They are supposed to arrive tomorrow," Maku nonchalantly reported. I was dumbstruck. Yes, there was still the myth out there that spinal taps killed patients, even though it was total rubbish. Ten years ago, when skeletal AIDS patients would be carried in with severe meningitis and would have a tap done, some of them would later die, despite the last-minute treatment given for their brain infection, thus contributing to the false rumor that spinal taps killed people. I recalled the struggles that would result when families adamantly insisted that their comatose loved ones should not get a spinal tap. But in this case the family wasn't there to interfere with the patient's medical care. I took a firmer tone.

"You must not wait for the family to come, you must do the spinal tap immediately. By any standard of medical care and ethics, you have a duty as a doctor to do what you think is best for this man and not wait for his family, who might not show up before he dies from whatever's going on. Please do the spinal tap, and you can document that I authorized it. Now let's quickly see the remaining patients so you can take care of these matters." We moved on to the female room, where the litany of neglect continued to unfold.

A 46-year-old woman was in for yet more blood transfusions for severe, recurrent anemia. I quickly learned from her that she had heavy periods, and on my exam there were large uterine fibroids—it was obvious Maku had never examined her. A 30-year-old woman, HIV-negative, had been on TB treatment for several months, but continued to lose weight, even though her other TB symptoms—cough, fevers, night sweats—had improved. It took me just a few questions to learn that she had recently been seen at the gynecology clinic at Marina and had been told she had "a problem down there." She added that she had another gynecology appointment in five months for this problem. Without prompting, she turned to her bedside stand and pulled out of the drawer a folder containing her outpatient medical cards, which Maku apparently hadn't bothered to look at. There, in plain view, was a pathology report which showed that a biopsy done six months previously showed invasive cancer of the cervix. And, sure enough, the people in Marina's gynecology clinic had scheduled her for surgery in five months, assuming she was still alive.

By then, I had lost all patience and commanded that the two women be sent to Marina as soon as possible.

"They will go, doctor," replied the nurse, looking askance at Machu. Thank God for Batswana nurses. "The matron will let you know if there are problems." Dr. Maku knew he'd better follow through: hospital matrons didn't put up with any nonsense.

I headed to the clinic, where I was supposed to see only patients specially selected for us "august" specialists. But today, as with past outreach visits, I would function essentially as a skivvy, seeing all comers. The clinic's waiting area was full, the narrow benches crowded with patients. The same grungy dog who had greeted us first thing had returned, as dogs are wont to do, warily slinking about, on the lookout for food and any ill-tempered nurse who might shoo it out. After knocking on several doors, I finally found the nurse who would work with me—Rachel, a heavyset, friendly lady, probably in her early forties, who happily identified herself as one of my KITSO attendees from many years ago. She seemed genuinely pleased to help me. Most of the nurses out in the boondocks were good, and, like the one on the inpatient ward, actually seemed to care about the patients. Maybe it was the small-town mentality, where everyone knew everyone else.

The procession of patients seemed to exemplify the successes and failures of the National Treatment Programme, as well as many of the Programme's trade-offs and risks. A 23-year-old woman, on ARVs for many years and doing well from the HIV standpoint, came in for routine monitoring of the blood thinner she had been taking for an artificial heart valve inserted in South Africa ten years previously, at great expense to the country. So many young adults here had damaged heart valves from untreated childhood rheumatic fever, and Botswana had given them many extra years of life by sending them south for heart surgery. One of the cardinal precepts of treating such patients was that blood thinners were crucial to keep clots from forming on the metal heart valve, since they could break off and stroke out the patient.

"The doctor stopped her warfarin"—the blood thinner—"last month," Rachel reported. "The lab ran out of reagents to check her INR." The INR was a simple test to make sure the blood thinner was at the right dose. This was certainly in the top-ten list of stupid doctor decisions, akin to telling a patient to stop his blood pressure medicines because the blood pressure machine was broken.

"Can we do an INR today? Are the reagents in stock?"

"No, doctor. Maybe next week." Or next month or next year. Rachel was trying to be helpful, but I'd long since learned that in Botswana they'll never tell you it's hopeless.

"Okay, Rachel, I think we'd better restart her warfarin, even if we can't get her INR. I think the risks of not starting it, especially clotting up her heart valve, are far worse than starting it." Not only would a serious stroke wipe out the benefits of her expensive heart surgery, it would also make her survival from HIV seem a little pathetic. The patient seemed to understand what I was on about. Rachel and I reviewed the various precautions about warfarin with the patient, and sent her on her way. But because minor miracles did happen occasionally, I told her to come back in a month, to see if the INR reagents had arrived.

"And don't let anyone stop your warfarin without checking with me! See: my phone number is here, under my name." I motioned to my note in the patient's cards. "My daughter went to school with her," Rachel added as the young woman exited. "She's director of our church choir."

The patients waiting outside to be seen were perched on the edge of the benches, their eyes glued on the door of the exam room. They had probably been waiting since sunrise, and they were determined to be seen. No sooner did the door handle move to signal the exit of a patient than the next one in the queue would leap up—assuming they were strong enough to leap—and squeeze past the exiting patient, quickly plop down on the chair next to the desk, and dutifully hand me their medical cards. Most of the time, trying to decipher the scribblings on their cards—as in the States, most doctors here had atrocious handwriting—was akin to translating the Dead Sea Scrolls. But Rachel was usually able to tell me why the patient was there.

A twenty-two year-old woman four months into her pregnancy came in for refills of her epilepsy medicine. To my horror, I saw she was on sodium valproate, which was absolutely forbidden in pregnancy because it often caused fetal brain damage. A quick call to a pediatric colleague, and she was switched to a safer drug. I silently prayed that the baby's IQ would be spared.

Another young woman—Rachel later told me she was a secondary school teacher in the village—came in for refills of her blood pressure medicine. But she had a far more serious problem: acute leukemia, which was being treated in South Africa. Totally bald from the chemotherapy, she was probably one of the most cheerful and upbeat patients I've ever met. She must have known how bleak her prognosis was—there was internet even in Hukuntsi—but she seemed at peace. I vowed never to forget her equanimity.

Next, a wild-eyed zombie straight out of *Night of the Living Dead*: I couldn't help myself, but that was my first thought when a skeletal twenty-seven-year-old woman with end-stage AIDS and TB staggered into the exam room, supported by her niece and aunt. The poor woman had recently been discharged from Marina. The niece and aunt said she was "much better" since leaving Marina. Considering her current state, it was probably a miracle that she made it out alive. She had that vacant, seemingly terrified stare of severe dementia—she seemed not to have a clue about what was going on—but fortunately her eyes didn't show any jaundice, which would have signified liver damage from her ARVs and TB drugs. I praised her relatives for taking her in and caring for her, although it probably would never have occurred to them not to look after her. "She is a nurse at a district clinic," volunteered Rachel. "I told her how ARVs had saved me and how she must be tested. But she feared her partner would abandon her if she tested positive." I didn't have the heart to ask if her partner had abandoned her now. "But God is good. Her family will take care of her."

A fifty-five-year-old man made me feel for a moment I was back in New York, examining an American patient who seemed engaged and interested in his hypertension and heart disease. As Rachel told me after he'd left, he was the manager of Spar, the supermarket chain that penetrated even into out-of-the-way hamlets like Hukuntsi. Dressed in a sports jacket and tie—as was the custom in Botswana, the manufacturer's label was left sewn on the out-side sleeve of the jacket and the wide tie hung way too short—he handed me a bound notebook containing his past clinic visits. It was opened to the pages on which he had written his weekly blood pressures, taken on his home blood pressure machine. All were perfect, not a digit over 130/90. As I wrote refills for his two blood pressure pills, I reviewed with him the reasons we wanted his pressures to be normal, patient education that many doctors didn't take time to give here. On the way out, he told Rachel he had set aside for her a box of fresh citrus that had just arrived from South Africa. He, too, understood that it was always good to have the nurses on your side.

As soon as the next patient started to enter—a young man who appeared weak and wilting—Rachel asked him to step back into the waiting area. Her tone with him was familiar, almost maternal. When another patient instantly tried to enter behind him, Rachel also told her to step back. She positioned herself firmly against the door to prevent other supplicants from barging in.

"Doctor, you do not need to see the next young man if you feel you cannot. He's a Zimbabwean and goes to our church, but he is not a citizen." I had already spied on her blouse a small star-shaped pin, which denoted her membership in the Zion Christian Church, the same church that Polite, my housekeeper from many years ago, had belonged to.

"So what do you think I'll say, Rachel?" I asked with a combination of jest, affection, and mock annoyance, slightly shrugging my shoulders with Italian-like ennui. Rachel was breaking the rules: except for TB, non-citizens weren't allowed to get any care, however minor, in government facilities. But she obviously answered to a higher authority. Moreover, Hukuntsi was a long way away from the Ministry of Health in Gaborone.

"Thank you, doctor." She opened the door and, beating off the other patients huddling outside, ushered in the young man. Instead of taking her chair beside me, she stood by the patient, hands clasped in front of her. She seemed worried.

As it turned out, Rachel had reason to be anxious. The guy, probably in his late twenties, had a bad outbreak of shingles, a sure sign of HIV infection. Rachel, of course, knew this. And she had broken another rule: she had done an HIV test on him, and it was, of course, positive.

Once Rachel's co-religionist—his name was Godwill—got out of his black leather jacket, the full extremity of his situation was apparent. I'd seen a lot worse, but Godwill was probably up in the top 10 percent of malnourished AIDS patients I'd cared for. His shingles cut a wide swathe across his left upper back. It hurt just to look at the red, angry rash, which was seeping clear fluid. The pain from shingles can be deep and intense—think of a pinched nerve, only worse. But Godwill's terror at what was happening to him seemed far worse than his pain. And poor Rachel didn't seem all too calm either, gently rocking back and forth.

My brief history and physical exam was remarkable only for his shingles and the usual white thrush in his mouth. I reached over and put my hand on his forearm.

"Godwill, I'm very worried about your condition. You're not in any *immediate* danger,"—I felt I had to reassure him, although he could come down anytime with a whole host of terrible complications—"but we need to treat your shingles and get you on HIV medicines as soon as possible." First, he needed to be on high-dose acyclovir for the shingles, and cotrimoxazole to prevent the AIDS pneumonia. That's if he could afford them. Rachel could do only so much, and getting drugs from the hospital pharmacy for a non-citizen would be daunting. I quietly sighed and looked up at Rachel. I reached for the thick wad of pula notes in my back pocket.

"Rachel, how much do you think acyclovir and cotrimoxazole would cost at the chemist?"

"Doctor, thank you, but our church will take care of him. The man you just saw from Spar"—my "New York City patient" with well-controlled hypertension—"he will pay for the medicine." Praise the Lord: a network of Zionists looking after their own. "All we need is prescriptions from you. God is good!"

As I wrote out the prescriptions, Rachel told me how Godwill's uncle, a ZCC elder, was coming from Zimbabwe next Sunday to take him back home. "The church there will help him with his ARVs. I have told Godwill how God saved me from HIV and that He will save him." Godwill was looking down at the floor intently, his hands clasped as if in prayer.

Time for a quick lunch break. I found a small bench under a tree outside the inpatient wards and tucked into my packed lunch. That same mangy dog gingerly approached me, his long tail lazily swaying, barely off the ground. I threw him a piece of my muffin. I now had a new best friend. At a safe remove, a couple of goats watched us intently, hopeful for the refuse. Although it was not quite 2 p.m., the sunlight was already becoming golden, and shadows were beginning to lengthen. The winter solstice was next week. This was my most favorite time of year, when days would be in the upper sixties and nights dipping below forty degrees. The hour before sunset this time of year was transcendent: the autumnal glow seemed to suspend time, before turning into an orange-red sunset that quickly ushered in darkness. I thought back to the patients I'd seen on the wards that morning. Several would soon be making the long ride to Gaborone, alone and without any medical personnel, probably arriving at Marina long after I'd hit the sack later that evening. Although transfer to medicine at Marina was no guarantee of salvation, they probably had better chances there than here. If just one of them ended up being spared, those were still brilliant odds.

Rachel and I beavered away during the remaining hours of clinic. From the outset that morning, I made a point of explaining to her what I was doing with each patient, tossing out various titbits of medical information, treating her like a colleague, which, of course, she was. The nurses loved it when they were included in the conversation.

Most of the remaining patients had their own individual litany of woes. A twenty-year-old man had sustained severe brain damage from a car accident, and came in for refill of his epilepsy medicine. His mother had to help him walk in and sit down, and since he couldn't talk, she spoke for him. There was a profound sadness and resigned resolve in her face. Rachel told me he had been a medical student at the university before the accident. Then there was an eight-two-year-old man who was coming in for follow-up of a low blood count from his HIV disease. Frail and barely able to walk, he was accompanied by his sister, who was equally frail. Each of them was wrapped in a thick coarse blanket, draped around their shoulders, over their heavy overcoats. They tottered in, hunched over and arm in arm, each supporting the other. If one had faltered and fallen, the other would have piled on top. A thirty-seven-year-old woman with a stroke needed refill of her blood pressure medicines. She was severely paralyzed on her right side, and required her two daughters to help her walk. Although unable to talk, she was cheerful and nodded her thanks to me. Most of the patients had nothing, or next to nothing, compared with my past patients in New York. But there was no self-pity, no complaining.

It was a little past 4 p.m., and we were finished. Through the window, the winter shadows were now stretching very long, and the sunlight was glowing. To make it home before dark, we'd have to leave soon. I hadn't kept count of the number of patients we'd seen, but Rachel tallied twenty-four. Not a bad day. She really was one of the best nurses I'd worked with in a long time.

"Dr. Baxter, before you leave, could you do something for me?" Oh Lord, I knew it was too good to be true. What did she want? A loan? A job in the States?

"Could you please renew my blood pressure medicines? I have my cards, and I've listed the blood pressures I've had done here. They're all fine." I felt like a shit, a typical cynical New Yorker, never willing to look for the best in people.

"Rachel, I would be honored." Her patient cards confirmed her blood pressures to be excellent, and I also saw that her ARVs had boosted her last T-cell count to 670. This was one of the many silent success stories of the Treatment Programme, reminding me that the desperate souls I'd seen in the clinics and hospital wards were only part of the story, that many had already been spared over the years. I briefly touched her shoulder on the way out.

"God bless you, doctor. You will be in my prayers."

The other doctors were waiting for me at the entrance, and we climbed back into the hospital van, probably the same one that would be ferrying the ward patients to Marina later that evening. The sun was low in the sky as our airplane bumped along the dirt runway and lifted up over the fence—the same forlorn donkey was standing dumbly on the other side. Since it was winter, turbulent storms weren't a worry, and from 22,000 feet, the slanting rays of the waning sun tinged the cloud tops with a reddish-pink hue. I tried to nap, but I couldn't stop thinking about the patients I'd seen—and about Rachel, and her church. I wondered how many other nurses like Rachel were out there, quietly lifting up those who were in danger of being pulled down. She probably had helped far more people that I ever could.

I mused about the very first outreach visit I'd made to Mole-polole, years ago, when death was stalking so many here. Since then, Botswana's Treatment Programme had put nearly a hundred thousand on ARVs— people like Rachel. The statistics couldn't be argued with: nearly 95 percent of infected people eligible for treatment were on ARVs. But there were still the 5 percent, the lost, the "defaulters," the ones who for whatever reason were still falling through the cracks—like the pathetic man earlier in the day on the medical ward, covered in feces and just found to be positive. I recalled from my Sunday School days the parable of the shepherd who left his ninety-nine sheep to find and rescue the one that was lost. I knew that part of our job here was to go after the lost sheep.

A little over an hour later, we were approaching Gaborone, for most Batswana the "big city." It was always a nice feeling when the pilot lowered the airplane onto the runway. As we approached the terminal, a lone South African Airways propeller plane was slowly taxiing to the runway for what was probably its fifth and last jaunt down to Johannesburg for the day. The sun had set half an hour earlier, and its pink traces streaking the horizon's high cirrus clouds were rapidly fading as we scattered and disappeared into the chilly night.

# Chapter 17

# Holy Cross Hospice:
# Final Lessons

Although many things had changed during my four years away from Botswana, Holy Cross Hospice wasn't one of them. The only difference was the big metal sign posted at the entrance which listed dozens of past donors—embassies, businesses, aid organizations, and individuals, my name included. But despite the many donors, the place still limped by from payday to payday, still dependent on the last-minute kindness of friends and strangers.

Howard Moffat remained the guiding force behind it, providing medical care and trying to raise the small fortune necessary to convert it into a real, inpatient hospice, so terminal patients could receive 'round-the-clock end-of-life care. It was Howard's dream. He had submitted a master plan to the government for its approval—and hopefully financial support—but as often happens, it was languishing somewhere in the Ministry of Health. He also tirelessly sought aid from the banks and international agencies. When he and his wife finally left the country for good in late 2014, to be with his family in U.K., his dream had not been realized, but he continued to work on getting firm financial support for the Hospice.

Like Diana Dickenson's, Howard's life was beyond exemplary in his service to Botswana and its people.

Just as the physical aspects of the Hospice had not changed, so the patients likewise were the same: end-stage AIDS and cancer were the usual problems. Although the National Programme had spared tens of thousands, there were still many who, for myriad reasons, were hanging over the abyss. And as before, there were many we couldn't rescue, but a few we could actually help.

Precious M. ended up at the Hospice largely by accident. She had been living alone in a small single-room house in Old Naledi, Gaborone's slum. When Puso, one of the Hospice nurses, was there making a home visit to a patient with liver cancer, the patient's daughter told him about Precious, who lived across the alley. Seeing that she needed help, he arranged for her to be brought to the Hospice the next day, when I happened to be seeing patients.

On that first visit, as Puso helped her walk haltingly into the consultation room, I watched her impassively. I had seen it too many times before. She stumbled and almost fell, before slowly collapsing into the chair. Although the heat of an early summer was already upon us, she was wearing a heavy cotton overcoat, which hid the full extent of her severe malnutrition. The vacant gaze from her sunken eyes I had also seen too many times before. Advanced HIV disease can often dull the mind, although one of the wonders of ARV treatment is that the mind can return, including memories misplaced when HIV was ravaging the brain. I smiled and asked if she understood English. She looked up slowly and vacantly nodded in the affirmative. No smile, no indication she even knew what was going on.

Puso told me what little he knew about Precious—that she lived alone, had no partner or family in Gaborone, and had recently been discharged from Marina. Puso really wasn't a nurse, and was more like a glorified nurse's aide, as well as an interpreter. His monthly salary was meager, probably less than my weekly withdrawals from the ATMs for routine expenses. He was a young man, probably in his mid-twenties, who was unmarried and lived with relatives in Gaborone. His home village was far away, just next to the Namibian border. He had an innocent, pleasing manner, and he understood my sometimes droll sense of humor. Besides, the Batswana still respected old people like me. I had immediately taken a liking to him when we first met at the Hospice.

"Puso! Her cards! I need her cards!" I commanded with mock impatience, tapping my pen on the desk. He quickly searched through the plastic bag Precious had with her, and produced a half-dozen tattered medical cards, including her Marina discharge summary and one documenting her ongoing TB treatment.

The cards told Precious's story clearly enough, and with a stereotypical, depressing monotony I had also seen many times before. A month previously, she had been admitted to Marina for pneumonia, which was diagnosed as TB. She had previously never been tested for HIV, and her test on admission was positive. A T-cell count later returned very low at thirty-four. She was discharged to the local TB clinic, where, according to her TB card, she had been taking her medicines daily. Under "Discharge Plan," the Marina medical resident had also written, "Refer to local clinic for ARV initiation." But nowhere in Precious's medical cards was there any indication of visits to the local HIV clinic.

"Have you been to the HIV clinic yet?" Precious stared back blankly at me, and then slowly turned to Puso, who asked her the question in Setswana. A pause and then a slow shaking of the head in the negative.

"She has not," Puso replied confidently, always trying to be helpful, even when things were obvious. Big surprise, I sighed to myself, as we helped Precious out of her overcoat so I could examine her. Another one falls through the cracks.

It was impossible to tell who was at fault: the doctors at Marina when she was discharged, the HIV clinic—often patients who presented for care at the local HIV clinics were fobbed off or told to come back another time—or Precious herself, who might have forgotten the instructions given to her when she left the hospital. Regardless of what had happened, Precious was destined to die—soon—if she didn't get HIV treatment.

My examination of Precious was as I had expected. She was profoundly wasted, nearly skeletal—small wonder that she needed a heavy overcoat to warm her frail frame. She had thrush, and her lungs sounded junky, probably from the TB. Returning to her patient cards, I saw a possible problem: at Marina, her liver tests were moderately elevated. I quickly rechecked her eyes for yellowing that might indicate liver failure. None, thank God. I feared that Precious might be in a no-win situation: her liver might be too weak to tolerate ARVs, but she needed them as soon as possible if there was any chance of stopping her downward slide. She needed repeat blood work to check her liver before we could do anything for her. I wrote a brief note on her patient card while Puso helped her get dressed. Just the ordeal of partially disrobing for my exam had exhausted her. She looked even weaker than before. I turned to Puso, and again tapped my pen loudly on the desk, like a dotty old colonial wanting his pipe.

"Puso!" He knew the affection in my mock impatience.

"Yes, sir," he smiled good-naturedly.

"This patient needs our immediate attention." I shifted my gaze to Precious as I continued. "You must take her at once, no later than tomorrow, to the local clinic to have blood tests, and you must collect the results the next day and call me with them. This is very important." Precious seemed to understand what I was saying.

"Please explain to her"—although she understood English well enough, I wanted to be sure she knew what had to be done—"that she must be started on HIV treatment but we first need to check her blood tests. Tell her it's very important and that you'll take her there for the tests." Puso leaned towards Precious, and for the next five minutes he spoke to her in Setswana. He then turned to me.

"She understands. We will do it." Then I realized I had almost forgotten to ask her a very important question.

"Do you have enough food?" Although Botswana had never experienced famine, patients like Precious often did not have enough food, especially given the country's high rate of inflation and skyrocketing unemployment. Eyes sadly cast downwards, Precious shook her head in the negative.

Reflexively, I started to reach for my back pocket, where I always kept the obligatory wad of folded pula. A few hundred would buy several weeks of food. But then a painful memory of a patient catastrophe from many years back erupted forth and stayed my hand. It was Comfort. I almost shuddered at the thought of how my overly attentive ministrations and prideful hubris had contributed to her death in her home village.

"I have asked the social worker to get her a food basket," Puso volunteered. Botswana's "safety net" for patients like Precious was a monthly basket of tinned meat, flour, rice, maize, fruit, and a few vegetables, which might last for a week or so.

"Tell the social worker she must have a food basket. Let me know if there's a problem. And we're bringing her here every day for lunch, right?" The Hospice van ferried patients here Monday through Friday, primarily for the midday meal. Across the way, I could hear the two cooks already clanging away in the kitchen.

"Yes, sir. We will give her leftovers to take home with her today. And she will get the food basket."

I turned to Precious. "Listen, when Puso takes you to the clinic, please show them this note I wrote in your cards! It's very important! Puso, make sure the nurse reads this!" I pointed to the bottom of my note, where in block capital letters I begged"

"THIS PATIENT HAS TB AND NEWLY DIAGNOSED HIV WITH CD4 34. SHE MUST BE STARTED ON ARVs AS SOON AS POSSIBLE. PLEASE OBTAIN BASELINE BLOOD TESTS (FBC, RFTs, LFTs) AND SCHEDULE FOR INITIATION

AS SOON AS POSSIBLE. PLEASE CALL ME IF YOU HAVE QUESTIONS. THANKS"

I drew a box around the message and drew several big stars off to its side. Someone would have to be blind to miss it. After my signature, I printed my name and wrote my cellphone number. If there's a God, I thought to myself, maybe the nurse who reads this attended one of my KITSO classes.

"Do you have any questions?" Precious shook her head in the negative. "Puso, please collect the results of the blood tests and call me. And I want to see her next week, okay?" Puso smiled and nodded his agreement. Throughout the visit, Precious had not spoken a word and stared blankly at the floor most of the time. We helped her to her feet, and Puso led her to the patient lounge for lunch.

Two days later, Puso called me with the lab results. They were normal, or at least "normal" for a severely malnourished AIDS patient. Most important, her liver tests were OK. Puso had more good news.

"They will see her tomorrow to begin treatment." Maybe one of the nurses there remembered me from KITSO.

"You're taking her there, right?"

"Yes, I am taking her." Puso never seemed to be annoyed with my compulsive concerns about details. Many Batswana were probably amused at how, in a New York sort of way, I would worry and fret about things like trying to snatch an AIDS patient from impending death. It wasn't that they didn't care—rather, many believed that there was little, if anything, we could control when it came to the behemoth of AIDS. For them, it was largely in God's hands, not ours.

Over the ensuing days, I thought often about Precious, wasted and beaten down, her wisp of a body shrouded in a heavy overcoat. She should have been "just another" generic AIDS patient, but for some unknown reason—maybe her name, or maybe that she was abandoned and alone—I really wanted her to make it. Perhaps it was how she epitomized the doomed here in Botswana. That she had no apparent family was both bad and good: bad in that she had no one to care for her at home and help her take her ARVs, but good because she wouldn't be carried off to her home village to die, as had happened with Comfort. Together with my intense wish that Precious be spared, there was also a foreboding: I feared I would jinx her chances of surviving. The gods, the fates—whatever impassive entities capriciously spin the wheel of Life and Death—would punish my arrogance by taking Precious. Of course, I knew my fears were irrational. Yet the last time I had felt so deeply about a patient was thirteen years ago, with Comfort.

The next week, Puso again escorted Precious into the exam room. She looked the same, still vacantly staring at the floor. Included in her patient cards were the lab reports Puso had called me about, plus a note from the local HIV clinic. She had been started on Atripla, the standard first-line treatment here. I could barely contain my excitement.

"Precious, do you have your medicine with you?" She awoke from her reverie and clumsily struggled with her plastic bag, slowly fishing out the bottle of Atripla. It had been opened, and the seal broken.

"Have you started taking it?" A slow nod in the affirmative. "You have to take it every day at bedtime. Do you understand?" I tried hard not to talk to her as if she was a child. But if she was to have any chance, she had to take one pill every day.

"Yes, doctor." Her first words.

Slowly, I went over Atripla's side effects—it can sometimes cause vivid dreams, dizziness, confusion—but I reassured her that these symptoms were transient. One of the few blessings of HIV dementia was that the mind was often too far gone to notice these neurological side effects. As I spoke, she fixed her gaze on the pill bottle, which I held in my hand.

"Puso, please explain to her what I just said, and how she absolutely must take her medicine every day."

For what seemed like an eternity, Puso quietly spoke to her in Setswana, probably relaying ideas far more nuanced and attuned to her situation than my English could ever replicate.

"She understands, doctor."

Two weeks later, Precious looked weaker, more haggard. Like a starving little kitten that's just come in from the rain, I thought. Again, she said she was taking the Atripla and, again, Puso reviewed the importance of one hundred percent adherence. To my relief, her eyes were not yellow—it would have been a fatal sign that her liver couldn't take both the Atripla and TB drugs. Normally, the HIV clinic wouldn't recheck her blood so soon after initiation of the ARVs, but because of her past hepatitis, I asked Puso to take her to the clinic for blood work. As I wrote the lab request on her card, I worried I was tempting the fates by giving Precious extra-special care that she normally wouldn't receive if she were just seen at the HIV clinic as a regular patient. But I convinced myself that I was simply practicing what I thought was good medicine. A few days later, Puso called with the results: normal. I tried not to rejoice silently.

After many years of treating patients in Botswana, I'd come to realize that I could "save" no one, that the only person I might be able to save was myself—if I was lucky enough to finally know who I was. Years earlier, I had tried to save Comfort, but my selfish reasons had damned her. I had finally understood my friend Aaron's condemnation, "You should have never got involved." My over-zealous interventions for Comfort—the food, the special treatment, the inordinate attention—had had the opposite effect to what I'd intended.

A month later—it was right before the long Christmas break, when all of Botswana, including the Hospice, shut down for a month—I saw Precious again. I tried not to allow myself to believe it, but she looked stronger. For the first time, she kept eye contact with me. As she got up to leave—she didn't require Puso's help—I wished her a happy holiday. For the first time, she smiled back, broadly.

Over the Christmas holiday, when I would think about Precious, I concluded that regardless of what happened—even if she crashed and burned—she had been given several precious months, months that she could use to set things in order with her soul, if indeed that was necessary. Gradually, I let go of worrying about Precious, although when I gathered round my family's Christmas tree in Ohio, I wondered how she was spending her Christmas.

About a month after Christmas—as with most of the country, the Christmas tree and decorations were still in place—I saw her sitting in the Hospice dining room, chatting amiably with two other patients while knitting a purple-colored scarf. She looked much stronger, almost normal. She stood up when she saw me and smiled, extending her hand to shake mine. We exchanged pleasantries.

Five months after Precious's first visit to the Hospice, Puso brought her to see me. "We think she can be discharged from the Hospice." I always worried that Puso was too eager to discharge patients. But Precious did look healthy, her face even a bit chubby. I didn't want to discharge her—for selfish reasons only—but I knew that Hospice resources were limited, that there were others waiting for our care.

"Precious, if you ever have any problems, I want you to let Puso know. And in your cards is my cellphone, so you should call me if you have to." She smiled knowingly when I mentioned my phone number—like all of us would do, the Batswana read over the notes scribbled in their medical cards. She waved to both of us as she left the exam room. I felt relief that Precious was finally released from the curse of my worrying about her. I turned to Puso, who was standing by the door.

"Puso, you deserve as much credit as anyone for getting her better. You were the one who took her to the ARV clinic and made sure she took her ARVs. You did a lot of it."

"Yes, I know," he replied, smiling.

Puso said we had two new patients to see on home visits. Because the Hospice van had run out of gas—a common problem, especially at the end of the month—we set out in my car. The patients were in distant suburbs, on opposite sides of Gaborone and in fairly shabby areas. Not slums, but neighborhoods where the apartment buildings were falling apart prematurely, and the older houses were akin to the dilapidated homes in the Hospice's neighborhood. They were not areas even half-affluent Batswana or whites would live in.

When I asked what was wrong with the patients, Puso seemed distracted, and vaguely alluded to "some sort of cancer." Since he only had a diploma in health education from a small technical college, I didn't expect further elaboration of their diagnoses. Puso never talked much, but I still sensed uneasiness in his reply. According to the usual routine, he and one of the social workers had already visited the patients a few days earlier, to be sure they needed hospice care. So he already knew what we were about to see.

The first patient lived in Block 8, not far from the airport, in an isolated area not yet heavily populated, save for dowdy, low-end apartment buildings here and there. The second-floor apartment was in a small, run-down complex that probably had been built only five years earlier. The parking lot had potholes, and the steps in the out-door staircase were cracked and chipped. The two-bedroom apartment was sparsely furnished but neat, and because of the Easter break, it was overrun with what seemed like a dozen little kids, shouting and playing. The patient, fifty-nine years old, was bed-bound, but greeted us cordially when we walked in. His mother was sitting in a chair next to the bed. She shooed out four kids who were playing in a corner. A quick review of his patient cards indicated that the Marina oncology clinic had deemed his pancreatic cancer to be too far advanced for chemotherapy, and had referred him to the Hospice for palliative care. He was also on ARVs and was injecting himself with a twice-daily blood thinner for blood clots in his legs which had been diagnosed at the oncology clinic.

"I guess for once this isn't another Marina screw-up," I thought to myself as I went through the motions of examining him. Pancreatic cancer was extremely difficult to detect until it was advanced, and there were no good screening tests to catch it in its early stages. It was a terrible malignancy to die from.

The patient fitted the bill for terminal cancer: he was emaciated, with negligible muscle mass. His swollen belly protruded out of proportion to his bony chest and extremities. I asked after only the most important symptoms: he had no vomiting and only intermittent abdominal pain. His only other complaint was pain with injecting the blood thinner. His English was good—on the drive, Puso told me he had been a science teacher at a nearby secondary school. My exam of his heart and lungs was perfunctory—the traditional healers had their incantations, I had my stethoscope, both of them equally useless in situations like this. I gingerly checked his abdomen, since it didn't matter whether I could palpate the cancer. The man seemed calm and accepting.

"Puso, I know this nice man understands English, but I'd like you to ask him in Setswana what he knows about his diagnosis. I need to be sure he and his mother understand what's wrong with him." An animated, several-minute conversation was interspersed with English. The patient mentioned "cancer" several times, and his words "no treatment" made my job easier. Throughout the discussion, his mother quietly nodded in agreement, her face radiating calm acceptance. He and his mother knew he was dying. The oncology clinic had prescribed morphine for pain, and the patient had a few tablets left. He probably would need more as the cancer progressed.

I told him how to increase the morphine doses, including the mother in the discussion. Both of them understood. On his patient card, I wrote an order for more morphine, along with a plea to the pharmacist to allow a family member to pick it up, since the patient was bed-bound.

"If there's any problem with the morphine, have the clinic call me. My number's here on the card." Maybe because opioid addiction hadn't yet reached Botswana, the one thing that most of its clinics had in stock was morphine, and there usually weren't any problems getting prescriptions for it filled for patients like this.

"And you don't need to take your ARVs or the injections any more. Just the morphine. And don't worry if it makes you sleep a lot. If you have problems, let Puso know. I'll see you in a month." "Hopefully," I thought to myself, "you will die peacefully in your sleep before then." The man and mother thanked us, and we walked the gauntlet of children playing in the hallway and stairwell.

On the drive to the next patient, Puso seemed troubled. "This cancer, it's not good, not good at all." I absent-mindedly uttered a banal soporific about life and death. I should have been more sensitive, but I was anxious to finish home visits and get back to the hospital to check on some patients, and then go later to gym, always a priority for me.

The second patient was almost a carbon copy of the first. He lived deep in Tlokweng, on the way to the South African border. In the 1800s, the Tlokweng tribe owned vast swathes of land, mostly bush, which the British confiscated. Because of extensive mineral wealth later discovered in the area—platinum especially—the community had been in litigation with the government for years to get it back. Imagine Native Americans trying to take back Manhattan. The houses in the patient's neighborhood were spread out and very run-down, but most had satellite TV dishes on their roofs and mammoth SUVs parked in front. His house was shabbier than the first patient's dwelling, with roof gutters dangling off-kilter and pavement crumbling at the entranceway. The house was also much older, so you couldn't blame Chinese construction for its pathetic state—it was built long before China had targeted Africa for its mineral resources. In the front yard, two old dogs lay in the dusty shade of a beaten-up car which probably hadn't run for years. The patient's brother and two sons were there, waiting for us. Although the brother fitted in with the overall dilapidation, the sons were well dressed and well spoken, and their polished Mercedes and BMW seemed out of place. The patient's bedroom was in the garage, presumably converted to his final living space only recently. Except for the bed and a small table nearby, there were no other furnishings. As before, the patient, who was in his sixties, was bedridden, and he greeted us warmly when we entered.

His medical cards told the story: again, the oncology clinic had pronounced his metastatic colon cancer to be terminal. He had a colostomy, and had been discharged on morphine. Included in his medical cards were small color photographs of his cancer, taken at the time of the colonoscopy, when he had been admitted to Marina for bowel obstruction. His records confirmed what I'd suspected, that, unlike our pancreatic cancer patient, this was a case of a preventable cancer. A year earlier, he had gone to the local clinic for fatigue, was found to be very anemic, and was given iron tablets. No further evaluation was made to determine whether he was bleeding from his bowel, until he was admitted for bowel obstruction by his cancer. Colon cancer screening was rare here, especially for government patients.

The patient looked much like the first one, gaunt and malnourished, but also with his mind largely intact. He said his pain was well controlled with the morphine. I went through the motions of examining him, and, as with our first patient, I advised him to increase his morphine dose as needed, also ordering more and asking the clinic to give it to a family member due to his condition. With Puso as interpreter, I verified that he and his family also understood his prognosis. Another easy case of terminal cancer. My other instructions, especially to call if there were problems, were identical. But I did tell his brother and sons that they needed to be checked for colon cancer, since it was hereditary. I told them I'd be back in a month, but I doubted if I would have to.

On the drive back to the Hospice, Puso seemed even more alarmed, quietly staring at the dashboard. "This cancer . . . it's bad . . . very bad." His brows were knitted in worry.

I was struck by his concern, since we had seen far worse patients with advanced AIDS, abandoned by partners and family, their minds gone, and suffering all sorts of serious infections. Maybe he felt protected from getting HIV—although in his mid-twenties, he always seemed very inexperienced and naive. But then I realized that I was being unfair to my young nurse: he had seen far more suffering at the Hospice than most Americans ever see in a lifetime, including on the TV and in movies. But for whatever reason, our two patients had laid bare his fear about dying, or at least dying from cancer, which, unlike HIV, was something he might not be able to avoid so easily.

I paused to consider my reply, trying to find words both to reassure him and to help him understand his own mortality. But I then realized it had taken me decades to reach my present equanimity about death. When I was his age—when I was a medical resident—I, too, had no clue about life and death, let alone who I was. Even though I had already seen death in my medical training, it was only fifteen years later, on my AIDS ward in New York City, when I began to relate my patients' suffering to my own impending mortality. How could I distil my insights into a few sentences to assuage Puso's anguish? In the past, I might have tried, but today I just couldn't. The forty-year age gulf between us seemed too great.

"Someday, Puso, you will realize that you will die, that someday there will be no more Puso. When and how you die really doesn't matter. What matters is that you live your life so you'll be ready when it comes." Puso continued to gaze at the dashboard. I suppose I could have appealed to his religious beliefs, since it would have been unlikely for him not to be a churchgoer. But I was too tired for such a cop-out. No, it was best that I say nothing and get back to the Hospice in time for lunch. Puso would have to figure things out himself, just as I had over my many years.

Concentrating on not hitting a herd of goats darting across the road, I then had a disquieting thought: had I really figured things out? Or was I deluding myself? In addition to preparing us for death (as Montaigne observed nearly five hundred years ago), one of the purposes of philosophy should be to facilitate self-knowledge. But the mind is facile in self-deception, constructing myths and half-truths that comfort us, at least for the time being, until death sneaks up and strips away our self-delusions.

I glanced at my hands on the steering wheel. Over recent years, they had withered and become the hands of an old man: wrinkled, less muscular, more wasted. It bothered me from time to time, but not too much. I accepted that I was getting older and that there was nothing I could do about it.

As we journeyed in silence to the Hospice, I recalled a dream I had had a few weeks earlier. It was actually more of a vision or reverie as I was falling asleep. I was very old and on my death-bed, and although in a fog, I sensed that my two beloved nieces, Katie and Maggie, were nearby. I knew I was dying. Because all of my siblings and close friends had gone before me, I felt very much alone, and my melancholy was acute. Maggie, a no-non-sense doctor, had just given me—either at my request or on her own initiative—a final sedative, and I quickly drifted towards my last breath. But right before the end, I felt a final glimmer of profound loss that I would no longer be among the living, that my life was over. And suddenly there was nothing. Just like that. At long last, I seemed to experience what my legions of dying patients had gone through.

As we entered Gaborone—lunch hour was at hand, and traffic, as usual, was slowing to a snail's pace—I smiled at the thought that perhaps God's little joke might be that I would experience death, the final learning experience, with terror, that my much-vaunted equanimity would evaporate as I was pulled down into non-existence. But no one would know, except for me. And no one would care.

We arrived at the Hospice just as the cooks were ladling out lunch. I wished Puso bon appetit and rushed off to Marina.

═══════

I really didn't know much about Eunice, who was sitting across the desk from me in the Hospice's consultation room. Spread out before us were her expired immigration papers and a government form that would ultimately determine whether she stayed well or succumbed to AIDS. Although uneducated, she knew their importance, and nervously focused her gaze on them, as if they might be a talisman or tarot cards foretelling her fate.

Eunice was Zimbabwean, and at the time in legal limbo. Her Botswana residency papers had expired several months before. Puso had given me an explanation as to how it really wasn't her fault, how her travels back and forth to her family in Zimbabwe had somehow caused her residency permit here to lapse. But I really wasn't interested in the details. Probably in her fifties but appearing much older, she had previously worked as a maid for an elderly Canadian couple, but when she fell ill from AIDS six months ago, they let her go, an all-too-common occurrence here. To be fair, the Canadians had initially taken her to their private doctor, who prescribed HIV drugs. But their beneficence for their worker of many decades was quickly exhausted, and they turned to the Hospice for help, since, as a non-citizen, Eunice couldn't get care at the government clinics. Probably because the couple were long-time parishioners at Holy Cross Cathedral, the Hospice took Eunice on board, and for several months it had been paying for her medicine, about four hundred pula, or forty dollars, a month. No longer allowed to live with the Canadians—they quickly replaced her—she had been sharing accommodation with someone from her church. In Botswana,

Eunice had two strikes against her: she was Zimbabwean and she was HIV-positive. Actually, three, if you count her being a woman. Add abject poverty and no job, and the impossibilities of her situation multiplied further. The Hospice was her only hope.

Eunice's situation was not unique. Foreign nationals, whether here legally or illegally, were ineligible for medical care in the clinics. If they ended up hospitalized, they had to pay upfront the costs of any X-rays, blood tests, and medications. The only exception was if they had TB—its public health risks justified treatment for everyone infected. But everything else was out of pocket—cash or no care. The government's reasons were clear enough: if medical care were free, as it was for its citizens, the steady stream of illegal immigrants from poorer neighboring countries, especially Zimbabwe, would become a flood of biblical scale. But at Marina Hospital, where every week or so a Zimbabwean would be admitted for complications of AIDS, it was difficult trying to treat a very sick patient who couldn't afford the X-rays, CT scans, and blood tests necessary to diagnose their conditions, plus the cost of any medications. More often than not, the best we could do was give them bus fare for a one-way ticket back home, where they'd probably die. The medical care in Zimbabwe was much worse than any place in Botswana.

The situation was even more dire for HIV-infected foreigners imprisoned in Botswana's jails and prisons. In 2014, two HIV-positive Zimbabwean prisoners sued to be given HIV drugs. When BONELA, a local human rights organization and a constant thorn in the government's side, won the case in the High Court, the government refused to enforce the ruling while they strategized how to make an appeal. Imagine the US Department of Justice flouting an order from the Supreme Court. Moreover, as a member of the Southern African Development Community, Botswana was obliged to provide such medical treatment to prisoners who were foreign nationals. As elsewhere in Africa, the government was selective in what laws and court orders it obeyed, especially when it involved HIV and outsiders, especially Zimbabweans. One of the legacies of the British was an arcane, byzantine legal system that allowed lawyers to delay, prevaricate, procrastinate, appeal and re-appeal, re-litigate, re-re-litigate, and otherwise thumb their noses at High Court rulings, especially if the government had decided to ignore its judgments. Government lawyers, as they often are else-where, were highly skilled at delay, obfuscation, and interminable appeals.

Zimbabweans were generally regarded here as leeches, taking up Batswana jobs. Worse, they were classified as potential criminals, guilty until proven innocent. Whenever there was an armed break-in of an upscale house or a brazen, broad-daylight hold-up at a busy restaurant, blame was automatically placed on South Africans and Zimbabweans. Ever since President Mugabe had reduced his coun-try to a basket case, Botswana and Zimbabwe suffered very poor relations. Police would regularly round up illegals, primarily target-ing businesses with day laborers. Those without proper papers were arrested and shipped across the border. My own experiences with Zimbabweans was completely at odds with the prejudiced stereo-type many people here had.

Today at the Hospice, Eunice needed a residency permit so she could return to Botswana whenever she visited her family in Zimbabwe. If she couldn't re-enter Botswana, legally at least, she couldn't get her ARVs from the Hospice. I had seen her only once before, when she first became a Hospice patient after starting her HIV medicines. She needed blood tests then to verify that the drugs were working, but neither she nor the Hospice could afford them. I paid for the tests, which showed that her T-cells had passed above 200, the magic number that often separated the doomed from the spared. Today she seemed fine, certainly not as desperate as many Hospice patients. As before, she said little, and replied in the nega-tive when I asked if she was having any symptoms. A diminutive, withdrawn lady with rotting front teeth, she had coal-black skin, and was wearing a bright calico dress, her balding head covered by an equally colorful bandana.

I poured over her papers. There were several prior residency permits, yellow and fragile, from when she had been a housekeeper, as well as her worn but thankfully current Zimbabwean passport. Among the scattered documents was a recent letter from the Hospice's social worker attesting that she was under our care, and was in the process of renewing her residency permit. Hopefully, if she were stopped by the police, the Anglican diocesan letterhead might convince them to let her be, at least for a while. The immigration form I was expected to fill out was fairly brief. Several questions dealt with her mental capacity, using quaint terminology held over from the British many decades previously: "Is the applicant an imbecile?" "Is the applicant a moron?" and "Is the applicant a cretin?" Probably somewhere in government statutes there was detailed description of what differentiated an imbecile, a moron, or a cretin, but I knew she was none of the above.

Towards the bottom of Eunice's form was a more serious question, highlighted in bold print and underlined: "Has the applicant ever tested positive for the HIV virus?" Yes, AIDS apartheid. Since her last residency permit, she had come down with AIDS. Until recently, it had not been illegal to discriminate against citizens— *citizens*—who were HIV-positive, and even though an anti-discrimination law was now on the books, it didn't pertain to non-citizens like Eunice. Answering this question in the affirmative would sink her chances of a residency permit and continued access to her HIV medicines. Maybe I was imagining it, but I felt the intensity of her stare on my hand, my pen poised over two boxes marked "Yes" and "No." Beneath this last question, right above the signature line, was the Physician Attestation Statement which ended with an ominous warning, capitalized and again in bold print: "FAILURE TO ANSWER ALL QUESTIONS TRUTHFULLY IS PUNISHABLE BY LAW."

Annoyed, I leaned back and stared blankly at the paper. It had been an excruciatingly hard morning of rounds at the hospital, and I relished the chance to put my brain on hold for a few seconds. A warm breeze rustled the window curtains. Birds were singing outside, and a red-eyed dove softly hooted from a nearby tree. Puso was sitting in a corner, perusing messages on his cellphone. In the distance, probably arriving from Johannesburg, a propeller plane, likely filled with businessmen and tourists, lazily droned on its final descent to the airport. I briefly wondered if it was Air Botswana or South African Airways. I sighed again and took a deep, meditative breath. I refocused on the form, hesitated briefly, and then ticked one of the two boxes. I signed the form with a flourish, adding my cell number and credentials as a Specialist Physician and Lecturer at the School of Medicine. The Batswana, especially the bureaucrats, were impressed by titles, and the University of Botswana was especially respected. Gathering her paperwork into a crumpled envelope, Eunice got up and left, saying nothing and not stopping to review the completed immigration form.

"The social worker will take her to Immigration on Monday," Puso volunteered.

Several weeks later, Puso told me that Eunice's residency permit had been approved for another two years.

We do what we can do, what we have to do—one life at a time.

# Chapter 18

# Princess Marina, II

When I worked in Iowa in the 1980s, one of my colleagues—an orthopedic surgeon and a nice guy—once quipped, "Medicine would be one hundred percent if it weren't for being on call." Being "on call" for emergencies, hospital admissions, consultations, or whatever was where medicine was a profession, and not just another nine-to-five job. On call meant your gym workout, your dinner, a movie, your sleep, or hot sex could be interrupted without notice, as you would be obliged to talk on the phone to a patient or nurse or another doctor about a real or imagined problem, or schlep to the hospital in the wee hours to see a patient with chest pain, or otherwise be required to do your doctor thing outside normal working hours. On call was what justified your generous income and high social status.

I have always hated being on call. Nonetheless—and here I blame my mother and Dr. Charles Carpenter—I always took call very seriously, sometimes too seriously. Carpenter, who was the Chief of Medicine at Case Western during my internship and residency, gave me my "medical conscience." He taught me that patients had to come first, which, of course, they should and did. My mother gave me primal guilt, plus the precept that the world was not a safe place. It was a lethal combination. My biggest fear about call would be that I'd mess up, that I'd hurt or kill a patient by not taking their concerns seriously. Yes, always a good fear for any doctor to have. An ancillary fear was that for some reason beyond my control—apropos Mother's stricture that the world wasn't a safe place—I couldn't be reached, maybe because of a phone problem or because I wouldn't hear it ring. Whenever I was on call, I'd sleep with the phone on the stand right next to me. I'd even take it into the bathroom.

Call at Marina for the medical interns and residents was as it had been since the beginning of time: they stayed in the hospital all night, admitting patients from Accident and Emergency and responding to previously admitted patients who were going south. By and large, they took their responsibilities seriously, although in the past there had been isolated instances of a doctor disappearing. Years ago there was a resident—he later became one of the specialists in medicine—who from time to time couldn't be found when he was on call. One night, the matron on duty had had enough and summoned the police, who hunted him down at his home and hauled him back to Marina. Maybe Marina doctors by and large stayed in the hospital because the nurses knew where they lived.

During daytime hours, the medical specialist on call would be asked to consult on inpatients on the other clinical services at Marina, which meant you'd have to go to their ward on surgery or gynecology or wherever, and evaluate them and then make your recommendations. Although always annoyed about being on call—it was a mindset I could never overcome—I really didn't object to seeing patients on other services at Marina, because the visit would usually be brief and I might actually be able to help the patient. If you thought the level of care on the medical wards was problematic, you hadn't seen anything until you saw some of the patients on the other services. Some of the on-call consultations were too sad to tell. Sometimes you wanted to cry or scream, or both.

One Monday when I was on call, I saw a patient on the neurosurgery ward, a fifty-eight year-old woman, a school teacher, who had been admitted a week before. She had been mugged, and sustained head injuries, including a jaw fracture. On admission, she had been awake and alert, and her head CT scan didn't show any brain damage. A few days after admission, a dentist saw her for her jaw fracture. The only thing he did—it was what catapulted the poor woman into the doomed—was to put her on injections of high-dose morphine for pain, to be given every four hours, around the clock, regardless. Now, whenever you give morphine, you need to monitor the patient to make sure you aren't knocking their lights out, as sometimes happens with heroin overdoses. And sadly for this lady, the nurses on the ward actually gave the morphine every four hours, as ordered. And as they gave it, the nurses dutifully wrote in their notes how the patient gradually slipped from being awake to then sleepy to then comatose. A few days later—it was a Friday—the neurosurgeons saw what was happening and stopped the morphine. I had to give them credit: they at least checked the medication order sheet. They even gave a few doses of naloxone, the antidote given for heroin overdoses. But she remained with the fairies. That was a Friday. Three days later, on Monday, they decided they needed to be more aggressive, and they asked me to see her. Talk about closing the barn doors when the cows had gotten out and were already beyond the border into Namibia. She was in a coma, with shallow and irregular respirations, and her kidneys were failing. I called the kidney specialist, but he didn't want to dialyze her. She died a few days later. I reported it to the head of medicine, but nothing happened.

One Christmas Eve—as usual, Gaborone was in holiday mode as thousands journeyed to their home villages—I saw a seventeen-year-old girl who had been on the orthopedic ward for many weeks.

She had a fever, and, apropos the old saying that to be an orthopedic surgeon you have to be as strong as an ox and half as smart, the doctor had no idea how to deal with it, other than blast her with broad-spectrum antibiotics. This, of course, was total rubbish, but what could I do? There she was, confined to her bed: a very sweet, very malnourished young girl with AIDS, who also had a very bad bone tumor eating away at her right knee. Probably out of compassion for her plight, the nurses had put her in one of the private rooms on the ward, and had even put up some Christmas tinsel over her bed. Her right knee was swollen to the size of a melon—the overlying skin was thin, shiny, and very warm—and the rest of the leg was also gargantuan. The swollen knee and leg were accentuated by the rest of her body, which was very wasted away. What pained me most was the total bewilderment and dismay on her face as she looked at her hideously deformed knee and leg. The nurse later told me that her mother and father had died, and that she had an aunt who sometimes visited her. I felt powerless to say or do anything to assuage her anguish, let alone tell her the "why" of her hopeless situation. As I was leaving, I wished her a happy Christmas—it pained me to do so, given the extremity of her situation, but not to do so would have been worse—and she smiled and said softly, "Yes, doctor, God is good."

After 4 or 5 p.m., you only got called if your team's resident, who was also on call that evening, had any questions about patients they were admitting. It was always a two-edged sword. On one hand, you really didn't want to be awakened out of a sound sleep, but, on the other hand, you were a doctor and needed to be available if required. One cardinal rule I always adhered to was never to criticize or discourage someone from calling me about a patient issue, even if it was trivial. You always had to modulate your tone, so as not to show annoyance. The last thing you wanted was a resident who was afraid to call you. Whenever I'd awake from an uninterrupted night of call, instead of rejoicing that I hadn't been called, I always worried that maybe there'd been a case where I should have been called but wasn't, or that my phone had been on the blink. Call it Carpenter-Mother anxiety-neurosis syndrome.

Once when I was a lowly intern at Case Western, we had a very sick patient with widely metastatic breast cancer. She was a private patient of what we interns would derisively call a "private slick." Her doctor was a pompous blowhard who always seemed more interested in his fancy cars than his patients. One night, the poor lady was tanking, and when I tried to call him to report her worsening condition, the answering service said he had an unlisted phone number and could not be reached. She died later that night, and the next day Dr. Carpenter stopped by to ask after the patient, whom he knew socially. Whenever "the tall man" appeared on the wards, always in a white coat, we interns always took pause, much the way a herd of antelope freezes whenever a lion saunters onto the scene, except that we couldn't race away. He was the son of a southern Baptist preacher and melded austere dedication to patient care with devotion to training his interns and residents to actually care about patients. I reviewed the case with him, and—thankfully—he seemed satisfied with our care. When I told him I couldn't reach her doctor because he had an unlisted number, Carpenter seemed genuinely confused, even dumbfounded.

"I don't understand," he said softly, speaking more to himself than to me, shaking his head in disbelief. "A doctor with an unlisted number? I don't understand." For him, it just didn't compute.

———

By the time I came on service at Marina, Isaac had already been a patient there for several months. Fourteen years old—the cut-off for adolescents admitted to the adult wards instead of pediatrics was twelve years—he was suffering from several complications of end-stage AIDS, including TB, KS, and profound malnutrition. He had been transferred to Marina from the district hospital in Tshabong, a small village at the edge of the Kalahari Desert. I had once taken a chartered flight to Tshabong, to provide "outreach" consultation at its small run-down hospital. Remote and dusty, Tshabong seemed to be at the end of the world. But to Isaac, it was home, the place he wanted to be most of all.

When I first saw Isaac with my ward team and asked him how he was feeling—like most young Batswana, he knew English quite well—he started crying, whimpering repeatedly, "I want to go home, I want to go home!" He ignored my other questions about various symptoms, and kept perseverating that he wanted to go home. According to the sparse notes in his chart, he had "failed multiple ARV regimens," and probably had highly resistant HIV. The reasons for his treatment failure were not known: perhaps the doctors in Tshabong were incompetent, or didn't provide adequate adherence education; maybe there were periodic shortages of ARVs at the hospital's clinic, an endemic problem throughout the country, especially in remote areas; or perhaps, as with many HIV-infected adolescents, Isaac just didn't want to take his drugs. No one will ever know how or why he ended up the way he had when I first saw him, bedridden, in a diaper, and weighing no more than 50 pounds. He simultaneously appeared much younger and much older than fourteen. His head was disproportionately large compared to the rest of his little body. His arms and legs were like thin sticks, small bones covered with skin. His prominent ribs had deep furrows between them. He was in a semi-fetal position, knees frozen in flexion contractures, as sometimes happens with elderly, bed-bound nursing-home patients. It had been a very, very long time since Isaac last stood on his own, let alone walked. And I knew that this little boy would never walk again.

As he continued to sob, I quickly did a cursory physical exam, going through the motions for the benefit of the four students bunched up around the bed. Turning to my team, which included a resident and an intern, I asked if they knew whether Isaac had any family—I had already concluded that the best thing we could do for him was get him home as soon as possible for terminal care. My resident reported that both of his parents were dead, and his only other family was an older sister in Tshabong and an uncle in Gaborone, neither of whom had ever been seen visiting him. That the sister had never visited was understandable, since it was a six-hour drive, and probably too costly for her. There was no cellphone contact for the sister listed in the chart.

"Does your sister have a cellphone"' I asked Isaac. He shook his head in the negative. In Botswana, one of the demarcations between routine poverty and extreme poverty was not having a cellphone.

"Does your uncle ever visit you? Can he take care of you, or take you to your sister's?" Again, a negative reply. "He works," Isaac sniffed through his tears, as if that explained the uncle's absence.

I turned back to my resident. "I assume there's no transport to Tshabong?" He confirmed there wasn't. One of the many problems at Marina was the lack of regular transport to the more remote hospitals, and on the wards there often were a handful of patients who could be discharged but who had to languish on the hospital wards, waiting until a hospital van from their particular outlying town or village showed up at Marina, usually to transfer a patient from the hinterlands to Botswana's referral hospital. The van would then return to the outlying village with whatever patients needed to return home. It could be a very long time before any transport from Tshabong showed up.

Like a few other attending doctors at Marina, I had forked out the pula needed to get patients like Isaac home by bus or kombi, but someone would have to accompany him on the trip to Tshabong. And it wasn't clear if he even had a home to return to, whether his sister would be able to care for him. Yet Isaac's predicament wasn't unique on the Marina wards that day, and having determined he wasn't in any pain or other distress, I had to move rounds forward, to the next patient and his or her own universe of woes. But, first, perfunctory reassurance to my fourteen-year-old.

"Listen, Isaac," I said as I leaned over and gently stroked his head, which sported a tuft of dirty blond hair, "we'll try to get you home, but it might take a while. But I promise we'll try." As I spoke, I looked directly into his large sunken eyes. I sensed deep, profound awareness behind the dark pupils. I didn't ask him to be patient, aware of the gross absurdity of such an admonishment.

As we left his bed, he was still whimpering, "I want to go home, I want to go home . . ."

Over the next week, there really weren't any new developments with Isaac. He was on multiple drugs for his many AIDS-related conditions, some of which he'd take, some of which he'd refuse to take, some of which were out of stock, and some of which the nurses never got around to giving him. But in Isaac's case, it really didn't matter. All that concerned me was that he was comfortable, that he was not in pain.

After my first visit, Isaac no longer cried but always asked when he could go home. And I would always reply that I didn't know. On rounds, he never seemed afraid, never complained, and never asked about his condition or prognosis. Whereas I usually tried to discuss such things with adult patients who could understand them, I never felt the need to do so with Isaac. You really can't tell a fourteen-year-old he's dying from AIDS.

Isaac was a quiet boy, content to just lie in bed and doze off. There were no books, magazines, or toys on his bedside stand. Fortunately, his bed was next to a window and not wedged between the beds of other older patients in his ten-bed cubicle. The windows in the adult wards were always open—"to prevent the spread of TB," as the signs taped on the windows declared—and whatever breeze might be roused in the hot Botswana summer would hit Isaac first. It never occurred to me to stop by and spend extra time with him, to provide emotional support or to make a personal connection, as

I had often tried to do twenty years previously on my AIDS ward in New York. I knew that such gestures would only be for my own benefit, my own needs, and not really for Isaac. Although I cared about him, he was "just another" dying AIDS patient, who hadn't had a chance to live as many years as most of the other patients on the ward, but who also had lived many more years than the innumerable infants and much younger children who had already succumbed. All I could do was to be kind and caring on rounds, to try to keep him comfortable, and to send him home as soon as transport appeared.

A week into my two-week rotation, my resident reported that Isaac had taken a sudden turn for the worse: severe abdominal pain, with rebound tenderness. I assembled the team, and we went to his bedside. I asked him how he felt.

"It hurts," he softly replied with a tinge of worry. His abdomen, which had always been swollen, was now hugely distended, the overlying skin stretched to a shiny, waxy sheen. There were no bowel sounds, and the slightest palpation elicited severe tenderness. When I quickly raised my hands from his belly, he winced in pain, and started to sob. Isaac had probably developed acute peritonitis or a perforated bowel, either one a major emergency. Most likely, a section of bowel had become gangrenous, and intestinal contents were seeping into the peritoneum. If it was possible, he looked even worse than before: his feet and knees were grossly swollen from profound malnutrition, his blood pressure could not be measured, and his bony ribcage was retracting with quick, jerky movements from the pressure his bloated abdomen put on his lungs. There was the musky smell of stool—his diapers probably hadn't been changed for days. He no longer had the strength to brush off the vexatious flies alighting on his face.

As I rattled off orders for the team to record in the chart—intravenous fluids (if we could find a vein), antibiotics for peritonitis— I briefly thought of calling the surgeons, to repair his perforated bowel. But I quickly realized the folly of such an intervention. The surgeons would think we were joking, so dismal would be Isaac's chances of even getting out of the operating room alive. I paused and took in the full picture of our patient: Isaac looked like a poster child for the Sudanese famine, or the horrendous Biafra famine of the early 1970s, or any other world tragedy. To my disquiet, I realized that *I felt nothing*—no ethereal passages of Bach swirling in my head, no epiphanies of the wonder and uniqueness of every human being, no sense of privilege, or horror, in attending to another human being's demise. Nothing. Except possibly a numb sadness at the sight before me: yet another AIDS patient was dying at Marina. But I quickly ended my reverie, and zeroed in on what we had to do.

"Is morphine in stock?" I barked. The resident replied that it was. Fortunately, it was rare for Marina to run out of morphine. "Guys," I continued, out of Isaac's earshot, "I want him to get 5mg every four hours. It has to be a straight order, not prn [as needed] or else he won't get it." Ordering drugs on a "prn" basis at Marina was delusional. "You need to check to see if the nurses can give it subcutaneously"—I turned around to scan his body for any viable flesh that could be injected—"and, if not, then he needs to get 10mg orally." My resident had been through this drill before, when we had shared ward service many times in the past and had similarly dire situations.

"And before you knock off today, you must—I repeat, *must*—stop by to make sure he's received at least one dose of morphine, and you should sign out to the on-call intern to stop by this evening and make sure Isaac's comfortable and getting his morphine." And then a minor miracle: our intern, Blessed, spoke up and said he was on call that evening and would stop by several times. Although new, Blessed seemed engaged and caring, and I had immediately liked him. I knew Isaac was in good hands that evening.

I didn't have to worry about Isaac's "do not resuscitate" status, as I often did twenty years previously on my AIDS ward in New York, when state law had required me to resuscitate dying skeletons who didn't have a signed DNR in place—it was a legal imperative that had enraged me many times. The Batswana had a deep aversion to designating anyone a "do not resuscitate," but in my many months on Marina's wards, I had witnessed only one resuscitation, albeit a half-hearted one. Almost everyone died at Marina alone and unattended. The emergency resuscitation carts were pushed into distant corners, shrouded in heavy plastic covers overlaid with thick layers of dust and containing long-expired medications and supplies.

Later that day, at gym, where I was able to resuscitate myself from the existential angst of contemplating Isaac's suffering, I thought about stopping at Marina on the way home, to see if he was okay. But I realized that such a visit would be largely superfluous. He was in his own world now, hopefully dreaming about happier times in his home village. My intern would take care of him.

The next morning on rounds, when I asked how he was feeling, Isaac was—in his own words, or rather, the only word he uttered, slowly and deliberately—"better." He had been sleeping when we first arrived at his bedside, but was easily roused from his dreams. His abdomen was no longer like an overripe watermelon, and there was neither tenderness nor rebound when I gently examined him. His medication sheet showed that the nurses had been giving him the morphine, or at least had been charting that it had been given. As soon as I finished examining him, he fell back to sleep.

Wheeling around to the troops, I commanded, benignly, "Guys, *this is how I want him!*"

Before we could even see the next patient, the ward matron— a buxom middle-aged woman with impressive shoulder epaulettes signifying her august rank—accosted us, arms crossed authoritatively over her ample bosom. *"The nurse from Tshabong is here,"* she announced with solemn pride. A major miracle, the news we had been waiting for, but which we had feared would arrive too late. Some poor soul from Tshabong had been transported to Marina, and now Isaac could hitch a ride back, at least to the hospital there or possibly even to his sister's.

Standing behind the matron's wide girth was the nurse, a young Motswana, in his white nurse's smock and tight white pants. We crowded around him, giddy to see if he was real, and if he would take Isaac with him. He seemed happy for the attention, and I quickly sensed that he was a good guy. I asked when he was heading back, and if he knew the sister.

"I return tomorrow. I know the sister"—given the small size of the village, it would have been odd if he didn't—"she will take care of him."

"*Please, please, please* don't leave tomorrow without Isaac," I begged. He seemed amazed that I would think otherwise.

"I will take him," he replied in a declarative, matter-of-fact way. He then strode to Isaac's bedside, and started to chat amiably with him. My last image of Isaac was of him with the nurse, who was leaning over the bedrail, talking with him. The incongruity of the two of them—one muscular and robust, the other barely alive—was stark.

The next morning, I learned that Isaac had died overnight. Most likely, his death was unwitnessed, and he was found dead in bed in the morning. It wasn't too much to hope that he had gently drifted off in the silence of the ward, in the cool small hours of the early morning, as the nurses were asleep at the nursing station. I could have easily checked his file, to confirm my hopes about his death, but I realized that it would make no difference, and would largely be to assuage and gratify my own anxieties.

I did wonder, however, whether the nurse took his body back to Tshabong, or whether it remained unclaimed in the morgue.

━━━━━

In my prior jobs, the morning after being on call was a time of relief, of quiet celebration that the annoying demands of call were over, at least until the next time around. But at Marina, the day after being on call was when the real work started: you now had to see all of the new admissions your team had signed in the day (and night) before. And usually there were would be a lot, up to a dozen or more. If it wasn't for the high death rate, the ward congestion would have been even worse than it was.

Like Morning Report, you never knew what you'd find on rounds of the new admissions, although you could assume that most of them were HIV-positive, either previously known positives or—surprise!— positives diagnosed just a few hours earlier. One post-call day almost halfway through my sojourn at Marina was typical of most of them. It was a Friday, and just happened to be the thirty-ninth anniversary of my graduation from medical school. For some reason, I'd always remember that anniversary, May 18, 1975, when we medical students lost, so to speak, our virginity, when we actually became physicians, no longer pampered and spoiled or able to hide behind the excuse "I'm not a doctor, just a medical student."

So it was a Friday, and all of us were eager to get started so everyone could get the work done before the weekend. My resident said we had eleven new admissions, plus the eight patients already on our service, minus two who had died the night before. So a total of seventeen, unless another patient or two died before we got to them, which was not uncommon. Right after Morning Report, my resident quickly rounded up our team of students and an intern. My job was to try to keep rounds moving forward, to teach the whole lot of them a little bit of clinical medicine, and—from my perspective, the most important task— to make sure we provided the best care we could under the circumstances.

Today, post-call rounds did not have an auspicious start. Since most of the new admissions were on the female ward, we started there. As all of us gathered outside the High Dependency Unit, right across from the nursing station, to see the sickest ones first, a patient from HDU—a young woman, in her early twenties—got out of bed, calmly walked to the area in front of the nursing station, squatted down, and proceeded to urinate on the floor. She then promptly fell over into the puddle and had a generalized seizure. Even for Marina, this was something of a spectacle.

"She's one of our admissions," my resident helpfully announced as we rushed over to the patient, who was jerking violently. "Well, it's certainly a good way to be seen first, isn't it?" I replied playfully.

The first rule about treating a patient with a seizure is to step back and take a deep breath, observe it briefly—the type of seizure can sometimes locate its origin in the brain—and then tell yourself that it's the patient, not you, who is having the seizure. In other words, don't panic. Don't do something stupid like force a tongue blade or a spoon down the patient's throat in an ill-advised attempt to "keep the patient from swallowing her tongue." Firstly, have you ever heard of anyone ever swallowing their tongue? Although Oscar Wilde once observed that it's not so common, you just have to use common sense: make sure the patient isn't hurting herself (as in banging her head on a bedrail), turn her on her side so she doesn't puke down her windpipe, give oxygen, check her blood sugar, and, if the seizing doesn't stop, give intravenous diazepam (Valium).

Our patient, who I soon learned had cryptococcal meningitis— she had just tested HIV-positive a few hours earlier—had the decency to stop seizing before the nurses could give my intern the diazepam. We pulled her bed out of HDU, and with the help of one of the nearby housekeepers—God bless her, she was stout and strong—we hoisted her back into bed. The housekeeper then quickly mopped up the urine. As I said, if Marina was anything, it was clean. So our post-call rounds that Friday had commenced dramatically, though not as orderly as I'd have liked.

The lady with the meningitis and seizure settled down and started to wake up a bit. The resident told me she was a student at the university. She was a good teaching case for the students, since the possible causes of her seizure were many, and not just the fact that her brain was teeming with lethal fungi. An important aspect of treating cryptococcal meningitis in an AIDS patient was making sure the pressure in the brain was relieved with daily spinal taps. Since there were countless patients admitted to Marina with this infection, the doctors and students got lots of experience doing the taps. The risks of not keeping on top of patients like this young woman were more than just death, and more for the students' sake than anything else, I needed to drive home this point before moving on to the next patient.

"Guys," I intoned, rousing the students from their stupor, "let me tell you about two patients I'll never forget. I'd just started at Marina, and actually it was here in HDU. Two women had cryptococcal meningitis, and were in opposite beds." I motioned to the beds right beside us. "One's meningitis was being appropriately managed with daily spinal taps, and she gradually got better and was discharged. The other had been mismanaged before I came on service. The doctors hadn't done daily spinal taps for whatever reason. So she gradually worsened and by the time I saw her she was blind and deaf. And whatever mind she had was now mush. She was essentially a vegetable. I don't want that to happen to this lady, okay?" Nods of agreement. They'd probably fight over doing the spinal taps since they had to do a certain number in order to pass their rotation.

The next patient in HDU, a thirty-two-year-old woman, had been admitted the night before for vague abnormal behavior, as in wandering the neighborhood naked. She tested HIV-negative on this admission, and in the Accident and Emergency note there was passing mention of schizophrenia. Well nourished, she seemed awake, but couldn't give any history. As I tried to examine her—she was still in street clothes and couldn't cooperate—she had an odd twitching of her lower face, on the left side. I asked the resident what he thought of it.

"We think it's a psychogenic seizure. We've asked the psychiatrist to see her."

"Psychogenic." It's a term we doctors both like and deride. We like it whenever we think a patient has a psychogenic complaint or symptom, because it lets us off the hook: the patient's a loon, or squirrel, or whatever you want to call him, and he's making it up, it's all in his head. When I was a resident, we'd call them "turkeys." Yet a caring doctor must also realize that from the patient's perspective their ache or pain is real, and they are not "making it up." But in addition to compassion for a soul whose mental anguish is manifesting itself as medical symptoms, there is another reason to treat such patients with concern: as I had learned over the decades, often to my sorrow, "turkeys" can get sick, with real illnesses. And an important corollary is that when "turkeys" get sick, they *really* get sick. So the trick when you're dealing with "turkeys" is that you always have to be on guard whenever they come in with this or that vague complaint. If you are a good doctor, you can't just ascribe their belly pain or gas or headache to their "turkeyness." Otherwise, you—and the poor patient—could get burned.

So our thirty-two-year-old lady had been given a diagnosis of psychogenic seizures. It's tough to describe a psychogenic seizure, but they're one of those things that you usually know when you see them. Even though I couldn't pinpoint it, our patient's twitching just didn't seem psychogenic to me. As I started to share my concerns with the team, lo and behold she had a definite grand mal seizure, arching her back, stiffening and then jerking about, rattling and shaking the bed. We turned her on her side and positioned her so she didn't hit the bedrails. The intern rushed to the nursing station to fetch diazepam. But God had decided to grace us with yet another of his little jokes: no sooner did our lady start seizing than—and you cannot make this stuff up—the woman in the bed beside her also started seizing: grand mal, violently jerking in near-unison with our patient. It was, to say the least, a scene.

"Get more diazepam!" I commanded one of the students, who scurried off to the nursing station. Fortunately, the neighboring lady wasn't ours, and even more fortunately, her team had just then entered HDU and took over her care. They said she had some sort of brain tumor and had been seizing on and off for days, because there was a shortage of phenytoin, the main seizure med at Marian. Within a minute or so, both women had quietened down. That's the nice thing about most seizures: they almost always stop, usually quickly. When they don't—when they go on and on despite repeated diazepam—it's a medical emergency, since the brain can literally fry from the overexcitement.

"Well," I said, deadpan, to the team, "that was the worst case of psychogenic seizures I've ever seen. Are we having a special sale on seizures today? Have one and get two for free?" Our thirty-two-year-old with non-psychogenic seizures gradually woke up from her fit, but still couldn't give us any history. There was something about her which made me think we'd never figure out what was wrong with her. Moreover, I sensed she would be in Marina for weeks and weeks, without anything definite being found or done.

Our next new admission was also in HDU. During the seizures drama, I had briefly noticed her in the corner bed, and hoped that she wasn't ours. But she was. Fifty-one years old, HIV-positive, and on ARVs for many years with a near-normal T-cell count of 499, she'd been having a week of shortness of breath and chest pains. She was also a diabetic, and her outpatient cards showed that it hadn't been under control for years, if ever. She looked terrible, fighting for air as she sat perched on the edge of her bed, half slumped over, disheveled in her street clothes, a purple beret still cocked stylishly to the side of her head. She really couldn't talk—every ounce of her being was going into breathing—and her lungs sounded junky, obscuring her heart sounds. Her chest X-ray seemed odd: it didn't look like a classic pneumonia, but neither was it typical for heart failure. An ECG would have been nice, but, alas, there was no paper to run one. Her blood oxygen level was very low. My resident volunteered that she was a lecturer at the university, in political science.

Overnight, the resident had started her on antibiotics for pneumonia, but I was concerned that maybe her problem was heart failure, maybe even a heart attack, although the lack of an ECG made it impossible to tell. In an American hospital, she probably would have been admitted directly to ICU, but at Marina either the ICU was always full or the patient wasn't quite sick enough to convince the ICU doctor to allow her to get in. I decided we had nothing to lose by assuming she had heart failure, and rattled off to the team the medications she needed.

"And we need to come back and check her out when we're done with rounds." I had a very bad feeling about her.

Another admission, a sixty-eight-year-old woman, was dead in bed by the time we got to her. I don't think any of us rejoiced when something like this happened, but we doctors are only human, and having one less patient to deal with was never bad news. My resident said that she had metastatic lung cancer—she looked it—and was brought in short of breath. I told him I hoped he'd given her morphine for her breathlessness. His affirmative answer didn't sound too convincing, but maybe in the future he'd remember.

The remaining female admissions were pretty routine—at least they weren't seizing or on the verge of dying. A few of them—one with an uncomplicated pneumonia and another with a blood clot in her leg— even had a chance of eventually being discharged alive and well. We then set out to the male medical ward, just half a dozen steps from the female ward.

The first male admission was so generic, so typical—I must have seen scores of guys like him. Forty years old, he'd been having a cough and shortness of breath for several weeks. His chest X-ray showed upper lobe cavities and a bad pneumonia. Everything about him screamed TB. He had never tested for HIV until the previous night, when, no surprise, it returned positive. My resident had already started him on TB meds. The nurses had put him in the "TB room," a four-bedded room a decent distance from the rest of the ward, never mind that the other three patients, who may or may not have TB, would be exposed to their roommate's disease. But better to expose just three patients than the other nine in one of the ten-bed cubicles. Our patient was very thin, and his mouth was coated with the telltale thrush. He was still in his street clothes, which were very dirty and stained. He was pleasant and cooperative but had that goofy, imbecilic smile that as much as said, "Help me! My brain is being destroyed by HIV!" This guy nonetheless had a chance to get better and not leave Marina feet first. Probably the greatest challenge was to ensure that when he went home—if things went according to script, he'd be out in a week or so—he would get onto ARVs as soon as possible. As with many patients, the problem was that with his dementia, he wouldn't have a clue where to go to get his ARVs or how to take them. Discharging him on his own would be akin to dumping him in the middle of the Kalahari without food or water.

"Does he have family?" I asked. Family, or a devoted partner, would be his only salvation.

"He has a sister he lives with. She brought him in. She said she'd been trying to get him to come in, but he refused." Good news, a small but important step on the way to becoming one of the spared. For what was probably the thousandth time, I launched into my lecture about how someone needed to be sure he and his sister were referred to the local clinic for ARV treatment when he was sent home. I charged one of the medical students with the task, a quiet young woman who had impressed me with her concern for our patients.

Our next male admission was in the same TB room, even though he most likely didn't have TB. Sixty-six years old and HIV-negative, he had been readmitted for a bronchoscopy to evaluate the large mass in his right lung. He had been hospitalized a month previously for coughing up blood, and his chest CT scan showed that the mass was almost certainly cancer, while his bones were riddled with what undoubtedly were metastases. Because it took weeks to schedule a bronchoscopy, he was discharged home two weeks previously, to return for his bronchoscopy, which was slated for Monday, three days away. I scanned his past records, especially the CT report, which announced his imminent demise. The patient looked almost as bad as his CT scan—he was very wasted, but was still strong enough to sit up in bed and smile when we approached. I motioned to the team to step back from the bed with me.

"I have just one question: why are we doing a bronchoscopy on this man?" My resident seemed perplexed, perhaps because my tone was a bit testy. "I mean, this guy has metastatic cancer, and even if we get a tissue diagnosis, it will takes weeks to receive the results from South Africa, and then what are we going to offer him? Chemotherapy? Radiation therapy? What's the waiting time to be seen in the oncology clinic? Last time I checked for a patient at the Hospice, it was four months. This guy doesn't have four months. And bronchoscopies can be risky, especially in someone like this. Tell me, if he was your father, what would you do?" Blank looks from my resident, and then he perked up with what he thought was a good answer.

"Yes, I know what you're saying, Dr. Baxter. If he was my father, I would counsel against it, but the bronchoscopy is being done as *an academic exercise.*" My mind instantly jerked back forty years to an event in my internship that was forever seared on my brain, a seminal lesson that was smacked into me by a seemingly unlikely teacher at Case Western. Dr. Olof Pearson was a clinical researcher, investigating new treatments for breast cancer. He'd admit women who were some of the sickest patients we interns ever cared for—cancer spreading to brain, bones, and liver: real train wrecks. Never what I'd call touchy-feely, Pearson wasn't especially liked by the interns. Short, heavy, and bald, he was taciturn at best whenever he was your attending physician on the wards. One day on morning rounds, tired and bleary-eyed, I presented to him one of his patients I had admitted the night before, another sad woman with end-stage breast cancer. She was supposed to have the radiologists insert a catheter into her hepatic artery, to infuse her cancer-riddled liver with toxic chemotherapy. After I dutifully presented her case to Pearson and my ward colleagues, he asked me what the plan was for her.

"Well, she's scheduled for intrahepatic Adriamycin, but"—my mother always told me that my tongue would be my downfall –"if she were *my* mother, I would send her home for terminal care, to keep her comfortable." I really wasn't trying to sound smart-alecky. Pearson, as was his custom, was looking down at the floor distractedly as I presented the patient, but with my answer he looked up at me with righteous fury.

"Dr. Baxter, if you *ever* treat a patient any differently than you would a member of your family, you have no right to be a doctor!" Even forty years later, the pain—and absolute truth—of his tongue-lashing stings. It has been a signpost for me as a doctor, whenever I had to make difficult decisions or give patients and families tough advice. Not as indifferent to my resident's feelings as Pearson was to mine, I tried to be gentle but firm.

"Not a good answer, doctor." I then told my team my Ollie Pearson story—they liked my tales from ancient times, before they were born, when I was a lowly intern. We decided to cancel the bronchoscopy— another poor soul would fill his slot—and counsel the patient and family on his diagnosis and arrange for palliative care, which usually was just copious amounts of morphine.

Our third male admission was also pretty pathetic, right up there with our other sad admissions. Eighty-nine years-old and a frequent imbiber from the illegal still he operated in Old Naledi, he had recently been taking traditional medicines for some unknown ailment. Comatose, he looked beyond dreadful: heavily jaundiced, malnourished, gasping for breath, and very, very old. His admission tests showed he had advanced liver and kidney failure. The problem with the concoctions peddled by the traditional healers was that you never knew what was in them—herbs, teas, antifreeze, rubbing alcohol, crank-case oil, fertilizer, insecticides, booze, whatever. No quality control, no Food and Drug Administration approval: just unknown rubbish, accompanied by scary incantations, all for a generous fee.

"Well, it sounds as if he's had a good life," I mused, surveying our patient's carcass. I didn't even ask about his HIV status, since it really didn't matter. This guy was about to check out, and trying to treat his liver and kidney failure was pissing in the wind. Besides, we had far more salvageable patients to attend to. Huddling with the team away from the bed, I recommended comfort measures only, as well as alerting the family to expect the worst, which my resident said he had already done.

Just then, one of the nurses from the female ward hurried up to us, to report that the nurses were doing CPR—cardiopulmonary resuscitation—on our fifty-one year-old lady in HDU, the HIV-positive diabetic with shortness of breath, the political science lecturer. I knew it.

We rushed to the female ward. When we got there, three nurses were around the bed, one pumping on her chest, another trying to fit the breathing mask over her mouth to ventilate her lungs, and the third struggling to unlock the emergency crash cart, which looked very old. It was probably ages since it had last been used. I had to give the nurses credit: their CPR technique was excellent, except that the patient's heart wasn't responding. No pulse.

A little embarrassed that the nurses were performing what we should have been doing, I told the intern and resident to take over. In fact, this was the first CPR I'd taken part in since I'd arrived at Marina. Most patients were allowed to die unattended in their bed, but this poor lady must have arrested right in front of the staff, who probably felt they needed to do something.

"Even though we don't know what rhythm she's in"—no ECG paper—"we should shock her, in case she's in V-fib or -tach. It probably won't hurt and might help."

The nurse uncovered the defibrillator atop the crash cart, sending up a small plume of dust that had settled onto the plastic cover over the years. Electrode pads were placed on the chest, and the proper voltage was dialed up on the machine. Before pressing the buttons, I officiously announced—just as on TV—"Everybody away from the bed!" Buttons pressed. Nothing: no dramatic jerking of the patient to confirm that the shock had been delivered. I pressed again. Again, nothing.

"The machine is not charged," the nurse reported. "The battery is dead." I rushed over and checked—sure enough, it was dead. I shook my head, more with resignation than anger. "Okay, guys: keep pumping. Can I get epinephrine in an intra-cardiac needle?" The theory is that squishing a large dose of adrenaline into the heart might kick-start it. "There is no epinephrine or needle, doctor," the same nurse reported. This just wasn't our patient's day.

We went through the motions of chest compressions and bag-breathing for a while longer. I rotated the students between the two stations, so they could get some practice for future CPRs. Despite our furious ministrations, the patient continued to be dead, and after ten minutes we stopped.

We stood around the bed for a minute or two. It's always poor form when you pronounce someone dead and, yes, they come back to life. The patient looked at peace. Her little purple beret was still pinned stylishly to her head. Throughout CPR, a woman in an adjacent bed took in the violent medical last rites we were enacting. There was no privacy curtain, no way to shield her from the scene. She lay in bed with covers up to her face, her eyes staring in stark terror at the pummeling her neighbor was getting. Away from the bed, I quietly whispered to my team important advice.

"Guys, you must always be careful what you say in front of patients like this lady, both during CPR and afterwards. None of us knows, until we're in the same situation, whether patients can still hear things during the final minutes of transition. So always tread with respect."

Of course, it would be the last of God's dirty little jokes that when I breathed my last, I'd hear the nurse or doctor gazing on my corpse say something like, "God, this old fart hung on to the bitter end. Why can't some people just let go? What in God's name was he waiting for?" Perhaps for the meaning of it all.

At this point, it was almost 1 pm. We'd been soldiering on for nearly five hours, and we still had several more patients to see on the male ward. There were lots of chores for the team to do with all the patients we'd seen so far—blood draws, X-rays, spinal taps. I excused the resident and students, and with my intern in tow, we headed back to the male ward. I was hungry, but always was loathe to break for sustenance until I'd finished rounds.

One of our remaining patients had been admitted many weeks previously with kidney failure. The high number of kidney-failure patients here always amazed me. The causes were many: HIV, traditional medicines, diabetes, hypertension, and obstruction of the bladder. Most times, we never figured out why a patient's kidneys had stopped working. But with our sixty-five-year-old patient, we actually found the reason: his urine flow was partially blocked, probably from an enlarged prostate, and the back pressure was destroying his kidneys, so much so that he had to be put on hemodialysis, at least temporarily. It took over a week to get urology to see him—surgical subspecialties were notorious for fobbing off consult requests. When the urologist finally saw him, he blithely said we should discharge the patient and have him make an appointment for the urology clinic, never mind that such appointments would be four to six months in the future, long after our man's kidneys had rotted, consigning him to life-long hemodialysis. What was even worse was that as far as we knew, this guy could have a treatable prostate cancer causing the obstruction. So our patient was stuck. We were waiting for the superintendent's approval to send him to the urology clinic at one of the private hospitals, where he would be seen much sooner.

At that point, it was half past one—visiting hour—and patients' families were streaming in, many with food, some with small basins to wash their loved ones or their clothes. Already a few were quietly singing or praying at the bedside. Rounds finally ended, I asked my intern to call me later in the afternoon with an update of what was going on with our patients.

Around 5 p.m., while I was at the gym, my intern called. The eighty-nine-year-old bootlegger with dead kidneys and liver had gone to the Great Distillery in the Sky. But there was good news as well: the cryptococcal meningitis lady was now relieving herself in the patients' bathroom and not on the floor, and the weird patient with "psychogenic seizures" seemed a little more normal, although her family wasn't much help in telling us whether she had always been a so-called space cadet or if this was a new condition. And, miraculously, our sixty-five-year-old with damaged kidneys due to bladder obstruction had been approved for transfer to Gaborone Private Hospital. The intern said she knew the urologist and had already spoken to him about our man. Not bad for a day's work.

An hour or so later, driving past Marina from the gym on my way home, I thought about all of the patients there. Not just ours, but all of them, the ones languishing on other wards, the ones on life support in ICU, the ones on other medicine teams. This evening, as usual, the parking lot was practically empty, basking in the amber light of the setting sun. As I always did—it was a habit I'd got into—I crossed myself three times, an atheist's benediction, my silent acknowledgement of the suffering there. It was, of course, silly, but I felt it was the least I could do.

═════

I never did find out Dolly's real name. Nor did I learn much about her past before she died at age twenty in Marina, other than that she had been diagnosed with HIV at thirteen, after she was raped by her pastor. I'm not sure why my colleague, an infectious disease specialist from America, had included this titbit in her record of Dolly's medical problems. At the end of their two-week stints on the wards, some of the specialists would compose a brief summary of the patients on their service and forward it to the incoming specialist, an attempt at continuity of care which a few of us made. The information in these handovers was usually short and concise. The specialist who added "raped by her pastor at thirteen" as a coda to Dolly's medical conditions was anything but a bleeding heart—hard-assed, not suffering fools, and sharp-tongued would be better descriptions of her. But there it was on the handover list: diagnosed positive after she was raped by her pastor at age thirteen. At first, I didn't think too much about it.

On ward rounds, when I first laid eyes on her, Dolly looked much older than her twenty years. She was in the female ward's High Dependency Unit. For the three days she was alive on my watch, Dolly didn't seem to change her position in bed. Scrunched up on her side, she was comatose, with an oxygen mask and a nasogastric tube for giving medications for her TB meningitis. Although usually infecting the lungs, TB can target almost any organ, and infection of the brain was a particularly bad type of TB. Dolly didn't have much of an immune system to fight her TB—her T-cell count was very low. And to cap her plight, her kidneys had shut down. The nephrology specialist had been duly consulted a week earlier, and he politely declined the option of putting her on hemodialysis: medical futility, dismal prognosis, too sick to survive dialysis. What is more, Marina's hemodialysis unit was already chock-a-block full of desperate patients with kidney failure, but who had more hope than Dolly. Although never discussed, rationing of care was common.

As I examined her for the first time, my team watched passively at the foot of the bed. It was clear Dolly wasn't going to be there much longer. She had shallow, grunting respirations, and drops of perspiration streamed down her forehead. The irony was that she

appeared well nourished, even buxom. I could hear the wings of the
angels flapping over her bed. Raped by her pastor at thirteen, she
deserved to be lifted up, ferried to a better world. Before I left her
bedside, I discretely covered her exposed left breast.

Once again, I faced an impossible patient with impossible medical conditions in an impossible hospital setting. Or, rather, it was
Dolly who was facing this infinitude of impossibilities. As I dictated the progress note to the resident, I mentally ran through the
few options we had for her. Ideally, she should get another chest
X-ray, to determine if there was fluid in her lungs, or a collapsed
lung, which could be treated with a chest tube, thereby relieving
her labored respirations. But the hospital's portable X-ray machine
had been broken for an eternity, and there was no portable oxygen
for one of the students to take her to the X-ray department. Dolly's
lungs were completely on their own at that point. We needed to do
another spinal tap, to be sure there wasn't another infection in her
brain—AIDS patients can have several serious infections simultaneously. And a tap might relieve any increased pressure in her brain.
We should increase her intravenous fluids on the remote chance that
it might help her kidneys. Finally, we should check her blood tests,
to see if there were any treatable problems.

When I came to the last part of my dictation—the "Plan"—where
we listed what tests, treatments, and other interventions we would
be doing for Dolly, I stopped and asked the team what they thought
should be done. Blank stares. The students looked nervously in the
small medical handbooks they always kept in their coat pockets, as
if the answer could be found there. My intern and resident as well
looked clueless.

"Come on, guys, help me! You've seen her longer than I have.
This is my first day!" My entreaty was half serious and half joking.
Embarrassed blank stares. I really couldn't be annoyed with them,
since, I, too, was staring blankly at pitiful options. I proceeded
to dictate what little we could do: increase her intravenous fluids,

check her blood count and electrolytes, repeat her spinal tap. And then a final question, mostly to let us off the hook for her impending demise. There was a tinge of desperation in my voice.

"Does she have any family? Are they aware of the prognosis?" My resident sprang to life. "There are two aunts. They are trying to change her name. We have counselled them." Good news: the funereal crepe had been brought out. "Family counselling" at Marina was usually a formal affair. The family would be taken to a side room, usually the nurse's tearoom, and with a nurse present, the resident would solemnly discuss the case and prognosis. Once I had tried to counsel family members informally in a quiet corner of the hallway, but the nurse would have none of it: we had to go to a room and formally counsel them. My only problem with such counselling was that too often the family would be counselled, while the patient was left in limbo without any idea of what was going on. That there was no mention of Dolly's parents or siblings didn't faze me: it wasn't unusual for patients to lose much of their family early on, and I felt that she was lucky just to have some aunts. I didn't ask why they were trying to change her name, since many times patient names were butchered by the admissions department.

"All right," I continued, safely out of Dolly's earshot, "the major issue in this case is how we can keep the patient comfortable. There's not much else we can do at this point. Yes, her mind is probably gone and her kidneys are shot. But we have to assume that she can still feel pain, so let's give her 5 mg of morphine, say, once a shift. That should sedate her but not knock her lights out." The resident dutifully wrote the order in the chart. "And when you do the lumbar puncture, be careful not to curl her up too much. Respiratory arrest is a complication in patients like this."

As we moved on to our next patient in HDU—a woman with cryptococcal meningitis, complicated by deafness, blindness, and dementia—I wondered how Dolly had ended up in Marina. Raped by her pastor at thirteen: there was something horrendously painful, terminally tragic about this, the only personal thing I knew about her. How did this violation of trust affect her? Did her family know? Did they reject her, maybe even blame her? Did the pastor infect her, or vice versa? Was the pastor with a legitimate church here, or was he one of the many fly-by-night charlatans plaguing the country? Was she regarded as so-called "damaged goods" thereafter? Young girls weren't valued as much as their brothers, so it was likely that she faced an even more difficult life after the rape. I mulled these questions over as I examined the woman with fungal meningitis, an elementary school teacher, whose brain had also become mush, because she had never been tested for HIV until she was brought in by her family after a seizure.

Then I paused. I silently surveyed the other eight women in HDU, all *in extremis* one way or another. Many were comatose, most were very wasted, and only one looked even halfway alert and salvageable. I suddenly realized that Dolly's pain was not unique. It was not—sad to say—particularly special. It was no worse and no less than that of all the other sad cases before us that morning. Who knew what terrible stories these other patients might have, hidden within themselves, unknown to the rest of us? Abandonment by partners when the diagnosis of HIV was known. Rape, often by an infected partner, or a stranger, or, yes, even a church deacon. Condemnation by family and friends when HIV infection was revealed. Loss of jobs, with employers turning them out once they fell ill. Church friends' pitying solicitations for a sinner who was being punished for wicked behavior. Above all, guilt and shame, the two most powerful emotions burdening most HIV patients. Within the female HDU, not to mention the entire female ward, a universe of unimaginable woes lay unvoiced, unknown. If I had learned of all their stories—or just a little about each of them, like Dolly's rape—I could have gone mad.

Over the next two days, Dolly's condition didn't change much, although if it was to worsen any more, she'd be dead. Her spinal tap showed nothing new. Her blood count showed a severe anemia, but there hadn't been any blood in the blood bank for at least a week. But in Dolly's case, it really didn't matter, and the lack of blood for transfusion made my job a bit easier, since otherwise I'd have to decide whether to waste it on her, possibly depriving a more viable patient of blood. Other blood tests showed deterioration of her kidney function, but we couldn't get the most important electrolyte, her potassium, because the lab continued to have a shortage of the chemical reagent needed to run it. This stock-out was now into its fourth week. Not being able to monitor potassiums in very sick patients was like flying a 747 blindfolded and not knowing the altitude or amount of fuel left. But Dolly was really on autopilot anyway. As with many of our patients, we were just going through the motions of providing medical care, albeit in very, very slow motion. My appreciation of the suffering of all of my patients made me no longer pity her, or regard her adolescent rape as a wound making her special.

Later, on the third day of my ward service, I ran into my resident, who told me that Dolly had died an hour earlier. "But her aunts were able to change her name back to her real name before she died," he added. "Dolly was her name as a prostitute. She worked in a brothel in Mochudi," a village north of Gaborone. No smirking or salaciousness; just an interesting footnote.

Dolly a prostitute. The news hit me harder than I would have thought. Raped by her pastor, followed by becoming a sex worker. Prostitution was illegal in Botswana, but, as elsewhere in the world, countless men, including the good and the great, enjoyed themselves at quite affordable prices. It was sad what a mere fifty pula could get you. Years ago, proposals were put forth in parliament to make prostitution legal. The same motion was submitted every year thereafter, and every year the male MPs literally fell about laughing. Nervous laughter; guilty laugher; shit-eating-grin laughter. They weren't about to do anything that might increase the fees of their favorite ladies. The inside joke, though, was that the woman behind this annual motion, a low-level government worker, had been a courtesan for many of the MPs. She had died a few years previously, after a long illness.

Over the years, when I was having a solitary dinner at Bull and Bush, a long-time pub where expats often gathered, there would sometimes be "ladies," young and well dressed, nursing their Tabs and Diet Cokes at nearby tables, nonchalantly looking about for a man who would pay. One of them in past years could very well have been Dolly. I studiously avoided looking at them, the slightest glance being an invitation to join me. Attempts by the Ministry of Health to reach out to sex workers to get them HIV tested were, as with initiatives for gays and drug users, half-hearted and hampered by moralizing and intimidation.

As the days and weeks wore on, I often thought about Dolly and the anguish she undoubtedly had suffered. And I went back and forth pondering whether one person's pain was greater than another's. The question was very important to me, because I would eventually have to face the emotional challenge of once again providing medical care in the States, after my contract in Botswana expired and I returned for good. Demanding, entitled American patients who acted as if their problems—their pain and anguish—were exquisitely unique and special had always annoyed me. I was worried that the suffering I had witnessed in Botswana would make it impossible for me to practice medicine again in the States.

But as I daily witnessed suffering in Marina, I gradually realized that my previous attitude towards American patients was arrogant. Sure, in New York, my HIV patients would have support and resources unimaginable to someone like Dolly—case managers, mental health specialists, social workers, adherence nurses, food coupons, housing, and much more. But would the anguish of an HIV-infected former drug addict who feels depressed and thinks she needs Percocet for chronic back pain be any less than that of my patients in Botswana? Would a middle-aged gay man's anxiety neurosis about his acne be less significant than the psychic pain Dolly had endured? I wondered what Dolly would have said. If she was like most Batswana, I bet she would have been a lot more compassionate and understanding than I had been in the past for such patients.

Whatever Dolly's real name, she and her fellow sufferers have never left me. As I would later realize, my encounter with this unheralded "train wreck" of a patient had radically clarified my entire eight years in Botswana.

# Chapter 19

# Final Departure

Have you ever noticed how clouds are both constant and inconstant, how they seem as immovable as Gaborone's Kgale Hill—the tallest in the area—and as transient as an ice cube on hot pavement at the height of a Botswana summer? As a cloud aficionado, I've always been fascinated how, when I would gaze fixedly on a cloud formation, they would seem not to move an iota, but when I'd look away for a few seconds and then look back, their array had morphed into something completely different. Botswana clouds are especially fickle in this regard—for example, awesome, menacing thunderheads rapidly evaporate at sunset into flat shadows fading into the ether. The same phenomenon pertains to how time passes in Botswana—when you focus on it, its passage is glacial, but if you just live from second to second, in the moment, time whizzes past. Einstein's General Theory of Relativity would implode trying to analyze and understand Botswana's time-space continuum. I loved the way time passed quickly and slowly at the same time. So as the end of my two-year contract at the medical school was approaching, I simultaneously felt I'd been there forever and for just a few months.

I was a popular lecturer, not just because I focused on what was important for the students and residents to learn, but also because I didn't hold myself aloof. Too many lecturers were condescending to the students, and expected them to learn about rare diseases I certainly had never seen in my forty years as a doctor, probably because that was the way they were treated and taught as students. Most likely, the only reason many of my colleagues were sad to see me go was that they'd have to be on call more often.

But my students were different. When told I'd be leaving, many sighed, "All of the good specialists leave!" Then again, students are supposed to flatter their teachers, although I like to believe they meant it. The medical students were my real joy. One of the tests they had to pass at the end of the third and fourth years was a practical, "hands-on" exercise called an OSCE, an "objective structured clinical examination," held in the medical school. We lecturers would man a dozen or so stations of ECGs, X-rays, real patients with physical findings, and simulated, make-believe patients. Students would rotate to the stations every ten minutes and were graded by the faculty members assigned there. Once I was a simulated patient with chest pain, and the students had to take a targeted history and tell me their diagnosis and treatment. One of the female students, always demure but very accomplished on the hospital wards, did such a superb job that I broke the rules—we weren't supposed to say anything to them about their performance—and as she was getting up to go to the next station, I told her she was fantastic. As she walked past me, without turning, she quietly replied, "You taught me." For a teacher, it doesn't get any better than that.

In October of 2014, at the onset of another Botswana summer, I attended the graduation ceremony for the very first class of medical students, held in the university's massive stadium. It really was a historic occasion. Amid the many hundreds of other graduates from the university, I sat with the medical school class—they were absolutely delighted when they saw me, snapping selfies with me.

Within eyesight of the graduation ceremony was further proof of the government's commitment to its new medical school. To provide its students a proper venue for their clinical studies—Marina was too dysfunctional for anything other than bare-bones education—the government was in the final stages of building a new, shimmering "teaching hospital," a 450-bed edifice just ten minutes' walk from Marina. Seen from the air as you landed at the airport, its immensity was mouth-dropping—it dwarfed even the nearby National Stadium. Mightily did Howard Moffat, Marina's former superintendent, try to stop it, contending that improving Marina was the solution. Howard even wrote an impassioned letter to President Khama, who polled the Ministers of Finance, Health, and Education as to whether a new teaching hospital should be built: Finance said no way, while Health and Education said absolutely yes. The majority ruled, and costly consultancies and 5 billion pula later, it was finally built, the Chinese handing over the keys on Christmas Day, 2014, a few months after the first medical school graduation. The problem was that nobody seemed to know what to do with it, how to staff it, and when it would finally open. Four months after it was completed, the Ministries of Education and Health admitted that they really didn't know how to run a hospital and said a private company should be hired instead. And the clock was ticking for the warranties covering the expensive medical equipment gathering dust in the empty hallways and surgical suites. Two and a half years after construction, the teaching hospital was still empty. As with other white elephants in the country, it simply was not spoken about for years, as if it didn't exist. But in Botswana things eventually work out, and in 2018 it's supposed to open with great fanfare, and will be named after Botswana's second president, Quett Masire.

I could have renewed my contract with the medical school—the Acting Dean and I got along well. The two years there were probably the best ones of my entire medical career—whenever I'd say this, my colleagues always looked at me as if I was wearing my underwear on my head. But it really was my best time in medicine: I learned—or relearned—loads of inpatient medicine, as I proved to myself that even in my sixties I could still do it. But as with my first stint in Botswana, I knew when it was time to leave, this time probably for good. I wanted to return to my friends in New York. What is more, I had two little grandnephews in Ohio to attend to, with a third on the way. I wanted to grow old with my three boys, so that they'd eventually love me enough to cry at my funeral. And maybe, just maybe, their great-uncle might guide them in a small way to someday feel and respond to the suffering of others. Not a small hope.

But I also returned to New York with some trepidation. Being one of those crazy people who define themselves by their work, I wanted to practice until I dropped, or until they intervened and told me I was too dotty to treat patients any more. I had gladly accepted a job back at the Ryan Center, not an administrative one, but as a front-line doctor and teacher of HIV medicine. Could I do it, deal with patients for whom I had previously had nothing but disdain? I sensed that my two years at Marina had changed me in a profound way, but wasn't quite sure exactly how. I worried whether, after my intense experiences at Marina, I could treat patients back in New York.

Whenever I had ward duty at Marina, I always kept index cards for each patient on my service, making daily notes on rounds about the patient's condition, lab and X-ray results, and medications. It was the only way I could keep track of what was going on. Even when they were discharged or died, I'd keep them. A few nights before I left Botswana for good, in the quiet of my bedroom, I tore up the hundreds of cards I'd accumulated over the prior two years, musing whether this card or that was for someone among the doomed or the spared—spared, that is, for the time being. It was an existential purging that perhaps made sense only to me. I burned the shreds outside my apartment, a sort of last rites for my patients.

The last day of my job, I got up a little earlier so I could have some time alone on the wards before Morning Report. I knew the students and residents were planning a little going-away reception for me right after report, and then I needed to head to the airport. Walking from my apartment to my car, I was enveloped for the last time by the pinkish-golden glow of winter's impending sunrise, still twenty minutes away. At the opposite horizon, the dark slate-blue sky clung for a few more minutes of night. Gentle clouds of smoke wafting from nearby fireplaces scented the silent chill. In the distance, a red-eyed dove softly hooted. It was the same sound I had heard on my very first evening in Botswana nearly thirteen years earlier.

When I got to Marina, the male and female wards were still dark and very quiet. Much like the western sky, they, too, seemed to be holding onto the mystical night-time stillness that's characteristic of all hospitals just before sunrise ushers in the usual din and chaos. I proceeded slowly through the two wards. The night-shift nurses were at their stations, dozing off or reading magazines, and the patients were all in their beds. A handful of family members were at bedsides, quietly feeding or washing their loved ones, or just holding silent vigil. Off by a window, in the shadows of one of the cubicles in the female ward, a hulking young man was leaning over in a chair, praying at the foot of a patient's bed. He was holding in his hands a book, a Bible no doubt.

Oddly, I felt no wistfulness, no regret, as I strolled past beds that over the years I had huddled around with my teams, trying to make sense out of the indecipherable, to bring a semblance of order to the unrelenting disarray. Rather, my entire being seemed so much at peace, calm and rested. I had done the best I could.

After an abbreviated Morning Report, the residents presented me with a small, touristy gift—a framed map of Botswana on which the country's coins had been pasted. "Where are the two hundred pula notes?" I joked. Then I gave them both a benediction and a great commission—a moral and professional charge—that I hoped they would eventually understand in their own medical careers, albeit many, many years into the future. Most of them had heard the same words from me over the years, as we made our hospital rounds.

"The challenge of being a good doctor is actually caring about the patient. Yes, you need to know some medicine"—here I couldn't resist pounding into their heads one last time some of my major precepts, such as always treating a low blood potassium, or always getting an ECG on a new stroke patient—"but you must always realize that your patient is someone's beloved spouse or sibling or grandparent. You must someday reach the point where you feel a state of grace in treating a patient or attending to their death, where you can feel the preciousness of all life and apply it to your own, when you finally take away more about life—*your* life—than you can ever give back to your patients. Remember: the only life you can save is your own. All we do for our patients is give them precious extra time to save themselves." God bless them, they all seemed to listen to my final words, many of them smiling with affection, more than a few with tears.

"And when you finally reach the level of understanding I'm talking about, I will probably be long dead. But when you do, briefly think about me, the old bald, bearded man from the States."

Late that evening, as my British Airways 747 arched up from the runway at Johannesburg International, shuddering and roaring into the dark ether, I thought back to fifteen years earlier, when I had left the 2000 AIDS Conference in Durban, wondering whether I would ever return to Africa to treat people with AIDS. I knew I had come full circle, from naive altruism—which ultimately was clueless and dangerous arrogance—to a kind of "African fatalism," and finally to a greater understanding of our universal suffering.

A mere twenty minutes into the long trip up the continent, the video flight map showed that we were just to the east of Gaborone, the airplane icon on the screen rapidly scooting northwards, past my former home and my many patients. I felt very alone, profoundly sad.

My heart choked and I silently cried.

# Afterword

One of the things about living in Africa for a long time and then returning permanently to the States is that no one really wants to hear about your experiences as an expatriate. They'll politely pretend to be interested, but they really couldn't be bothered. Moreover, it was well-nigh impossible to describe what I had done in Botswana. Maybe if a camera crew had followed me on Marina rounds, my friends and family might understand. Otherwise, I had to grope for words to describe what I had been through.

As my departure from Botswana loomed, I worried over how I would handle returning to my old community health center, to care for America's demanding patients, for whom I had felt withering contempt for many years. St. Clare's was probably the last time I had enjoyed medicine in America, and that was largely in-patient, not out-patient as I'd be doing at the Ryan Center. On one hand, I felt that, compared with what I'd done in Botswana, anything I'd now do in the States would be second-rate and insubstantial. But I also sensed that I was a new person—indeed, a wholly different doctor—from the one I had been two years earlier, when I fled the insanity of American healthcare.

By the end of my first week back at Ryan, I knew that something indeed had happened: I genuinely enjoyed outpatient care as I never had in the past, even with those very few patients who were difficult to please. And my patients returned the love. No longer did I trivialize in my mind their seemingly minor ailments and complaints, no longer did I rate or prioritize their suffering in line with what I had witnessed in Botswana. I was able to feel and understand the anguish an inescapably obese patient had over her knee pain and depression, or the despair of a man with emphysema who continued to smoke despite his worsening shortness of breath.

What had happened in Botswana that caused this complete turnaround? Whenever I ask myself this question, I always think of Dolly, raped by her pastor at thirteen, dying from AIDS at twenty, and the almost out-of-body epiphany I had experienced as I contemplated her suffering. But it was much more than just this one, heart-breaking patient. Dolly was the tipping point, the last straw, if you will, but she was just one of countless patients with unfathomable woes whose lives had intersected with mine. There was Isaac, the fourteen-year-old pining for his home village as his life ebbed away—his suffering evoked both nothing and everything from me. And Precious, the Hospice patient about to be pulled under by AIDS, whom I really, really wanted to "save" and probably did. And Thapelo, the young university student gasping for air, whose suffering I must remember when my own time inevitably comes. And Rachel, the nurse at Hukuntsi, who was thriving on ARVs and shared her hope and optimism with her patients. And, of course, Comfort and Polite, my early failures.

Now, whenever I gaze on the waiting room at Ryan, full of so many patients with broken bodies and spirits, I feel the presence of my patients in Botswana, reminding me that no one's suffering is greater than anyone else's.

I now realize I had gone to Botswana in 2002 to validate my contempt for American patients, to feel superior to them. Africa laid bare my arrogance and cast me down, only to restore me gradually to greater knowledge about myself and my patients. I had seen my own heart of darkness, and had emerged from it a different person, a different doctor, finally able "to feel another's woe, to hide the fault I see."

I had also gone full circle in the sense that my career followed the awesome trajectory of the HIV epidemic: from the first distant reports of a strange, mysterious illness when I was in rural Iowa; to the chaos of the so-called "new face" of AIDS at St. Clare's; to becoming an "AIDS whore" at the Ryan Center; to my first hapless arrival in Botswana in 2002, when my hubris ruined several patients' lives; and, finally, to my foray into the belly of the beast at Marina Hospital, where I finally felt and comprehended the universality of our suffering.

Nowadays, researchers seriously talk about finding a "cure" for HIV, and in a few years it may indeed be found. Whether it will ever be affordable for Africans remains to be seen, but I remember when just ARV therapy was believed to be out of reach of most people on the continent. So it could happen even in Botswana. And when it does, the world can rejoice, though we must also never forget the great suffering that preceded it, the many stories of both the doomed and the spared.

CPSIA information can be obtained
at www.ICGtesting.com
Printed in the USA
FFOW03n0314130318
45623095-46427FF